AF289729

In memoriam Franz Gross

C. Steichele · U. Abshagen · J. Koch-Weser (eds.)

Drugs between Research and Regulations

With the collaboration of
D. Lorke, D. Reinhardt, B. Schnieders and N. Victor

Proceedings of the 5th International Meeting
of Pharmaceutical Physicians
Munich, October 14–17, 1984

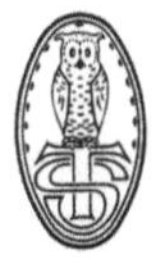

Springer-Verlag Berlin
Heidelberg GmbH

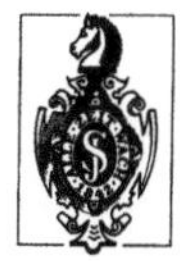

Steichele, Dr. med., C., Medizinischer Direktor,
ICI-Pharma Arzneimittelwerk Plankstadt, Postfach 10 31 09,
D-6900 Heidelberg, FRG

Abshagen, Prof. Dr. med., U., Leiter Produktentwicklung Therapeutica,
Boehringer Mannheim GmbH, Sandhofer Straße 116,
D-6800 Mannheim 31, FRG

Koch-Weser, J., M.D., Director of Clinical Research,
F. Hoffmann-La Roche & Co. Ltd., CH-4002 Basel,
Switzerland

CIP-Kurztitelaufnahme der Deutschen Bibliothek

Drugs between research and regulations : proceedings
of the 5th Internat. Meeting of Pharmaceut.
Physicians Munich, October 14–17, 1984 / C.
Steichele . . . (eds.). With the collab. of D.
Lorke . . .
   ISBN 978-3-642-54132-2   ISBN 978-3-642-54130-8 (eBook)
   DOI 10.1007/978-3-642-54130-8
NE: Steichele, Carl [Hrsg.]; International
Meeting of Pharmaceutical Physicians ⟨05, 1984,
München⟩

Preface

Franz Gross died suddenly during preparations for the meeting. He would have taken great pleasure in summarizing in this preface the aims and results of a gathering which so clearly bore his imprint as Chairman of the Scientific Program Committee. His sudden passing away is deeply regretted by all of us: organizers, speakers and participants. We greatly respect him for his exceptional abilities, his impact on science and his qualities as a human being. He provided the impulse for a well balanced and topical scientific program. We therefore dedicate the proceedings of this symposium to his memory.

Munich was the fifth in a traditional line of international meetings of pharmaceutical physicians held at three-year intervals, starting in London in 1972 ('International Aspects of Drug Evaluation and Usage'), and followed by Florence in 1975 ('Rationality of Drug Development'), Brussels in 1978 ('Pharmaceutical Medicine – the Future') and Paris in 1981 ('Drug Safety – Progress and Controversies').

This 5th meeting discussed improvements in drug development and application and examined the impact of regulatory activities.

Six sessions covered a broad range of topics:

hazard and risk assessment by chronic toxicity studies and the never-ending debate on the problems of their extrapolation to the human condition, including critical questions about the scientifically justified extent of regulatory requirements and about alternative approaches;

limitations of the significance of clinical trials for pharmacotherapy in the environment of general practice and possibilities of improving their informative value for the practising physician;

problems of the need as well as of the planning, financing, analysis and interpretation of long-term intervention and prevention studies including their impact on medicine;

new pragmatic biostatistical concepts for clinical trials and drug epidemiology;

problems of clinical trials in children, possible ways of improvement and ethical aspects;

and finally, discussions on registration procedures in Europe and the problems of international acceptance of data.

Interest continues to grow in the activities of the German Association of Pharmaceutical Physicians as organizer and of the International Federation of Associations of Pharmaceutical Physicians as sponsor. This proves the value of scientific meetings of pharmaceutical physicians in the professional world of pharmaceutical medicine and related areas. We hope that this 5th International Meeting has contributed to a strengthening of understanding and cooperation between doctors in the pharmaceutical industry, in universities, in hospitals and private practice as well as in health authorities throughout the world.

The Editors of the Proceedings of the 5th International Meeting of Pharmaceutical Physicians are greatly indebted to many individuals and associations both inside and outside the pharmaceutical industry. Particular acknowledgements are due to Drs. John Burke, Herman Lahon and Richard Rondel for their invaluable support in the development of the scientific program, as well as to Ingeborg Mohar, Frauke Kaluza, Ingrid Beyrow and Barbara Ritzert for their assistance in organizing the meeting. Special thanks are further due to Professor Hansgeorg Gareis and to the Paul Martini Foundation of the Association of Research-Based Pharmaceutical Companies (Paul-Martini-Stiftung der Medizinisch Pharmazeutischen Studiengesellschaft e.V.) and the German Society for Medical Documentation, Informatics and Statistics (Deutsche Gesellschaft für Medizinische Dokumentation, Informatik und Statistik e.V. – gmds) for permitting the inclusion in these proceedings of Professor Gareis' special lecture 'Research and Responsibilities' held to mark the occasion of the award of the Paul Martini Prize 1984.

Contents

VIII

Proceedings of the 5th International Meeting of Pharmaceutical Physicians, Munich, 14–17 October 1984

Chairman of the Congress
K.-J. Hahn, Ludwigshafen

Chairmen of the Sessions
D. Lorke, Wuppertal
J. Koch-Weser, Basle
K.-H. Breddin, Frankfurt
E. Marubini, Milan
S. J. Yaffe, Bethesda
D. Reinhardt, Düsseldorf
B. Schnieders, Berlin
D. Poggiolini, Rome

Scientific Program Committee
F. Gross †, Heidelberg
U. Abshagen, Mannheim
J. M. Fox, Cologne
M. Garnier, Munich
C. R. B. Joyce, Basle
H. Kleinsorge, Mainz
J. Koch-Weser, Basle
E. Schütz, Frankfurt
C. Steichele, Heidelberg
N. Victor, Heidelberg

Organizing Committee
C. Steichele, Heidelberg
K. Bestehorn, Bielefeld
H. D. Braun, Munich
K. Dolega, Munich
M. Garnier, Munich
H. J. Grigoleit, Frankfurt
S. Hiemstra, Munich
Th.-M. Kris, Munich

Contributors

Alexandre, J.-M., Professeur agrégé, Départment de Pharmacologie,
Hôpital Broussais, 96, rue Didot, F-75674 Paris Cedex 14, France

Baß, Dr. med., R., Institut für Arzneimittel des Bundesgesundheitsamtes,
Seestraße 10, D-1000 Berlin 65, FRG

Bilstad, James M., M.D., Deputy Director, Office of Biologics,
Research and Review, Center for Drugs and Biologics, Food and Drug
Administration, 5600 Fishers Lane, Rockville, Maryland 20857, USA

Boréus, Lars, O., M.D., Department of Clinical Pharmacology,
Karolinska Hospital, P.O. Box 60 500, S-104 01 Stockholm, Sweden

Breddin, Prof. Dr. med., K. H., Klinikum der Johann-Wolfgang-Goethe-Universität,
Zentrum der Inneren Medizin, Abteilung Angiologie,
Theodor-Stern-Kai 7, D-6000 Frankfurt 70, FRG

Deutsch, Prof. Dr. jur., E., Georg-August-Universität Göttingen,
Abteilung für Internationales und Ausländisches Privatrecht,
Nikolausbergweg 9 a, D-3400 Göttingen, FRG

Drews, Professor Dr. med., J., Sandoz AG,
Kohlenstrasse, CH-4002 Basel, Switzerland

Dukes, M. N. G., M.D., Regional Officer for Pharmaceuticals and Drug Utilization,
World Health Organisation, 8, Scherfigsvej, DK-2100 Copenhagen, Denmark

Epstein, Prof. Dr. med., Dr. h.c., F. H., Institut für Sozial- und Präventivmedizin,
Universität Zürich, Gloriastrasse 30, CH-8006 Zürich, for correspondence:
Lindenstrasse 37, CH-8008 Zürich, Switzerland

Fell, P. J., M.D., Deddington Health Centre,
Earls Lane, Oxfordshire OX5 4TQ, Great Britain

Fischer, Dr. iur. P., Direktor, Interkantonale Kontrollstelle für Heilmittel, Postfach,
Erlachstrasse 8, CH-3012 Bern, Switzerland

Fitzgerald, J. D., M.D., ICI PLC, Pharmaceuticals Division, Alderley Park,
Macclesfield Cheshire SK10 4TF, Great Britain

Fröhlich, Dr. med., E., Ciba-Geigy AG, Toxicology, CH-4002 Basel, Switzerland

Fülgraff, Prof. Dr. med., G., Staatssekretär a. D.,
Clausewitzstrasse 8, D-1000 Berlin 12, FRG

Gareis, Prof. Dr. rer. nat., H., Hoechst AG, Postfach 80 03 20, D-6230 Frankfurt 80,
FRG

Hahn, Prof. Dr. med., K.-J., Vorsitzender der Fachgesellschaft der Ärzte in der Pharmazeutischen Industrie e.V., Postfach 21 08 05, D-6700 Ludwigshafen, FRG

Heimann, Prof. Dr. med., G., Universitäts-Kinderklinik, Josef-Steltzmann-Strasse 9, D-5000 Köln 41, FRG

Hess, Prof. Dr. med., R., Stellvertretender Direktor, Ciba-Geigy AG, CH-4002 Basel, Switzerland

Joyce, C. R. B., M.D., Ciba-Geigy AG, Medical Dept., CH-4002 Basel, Switzerland

Krebs, Prof. Dr. med., R., Leiter Forschung und Entwicklung, Bayer AG, Forschungszentrum Wuppertal, Friedrich-Ebert-Strasse, D-5600 Wuppertal 1, FRG

Lasagna, M.D., L., Professor of Pharmacology, Tufts University, Boston, Mass. 02111, USA

Liebeswar, Univ.-Doz. Dr., G., Oberrat, Sektion Volksgesundheit, Bundesministerium für Gesundheit und Umweltschutz, Sektion II, Stubenring 1, A-1010 Wien, Austria

Lorke, Prof. Dr. med., D., Leiter des Instituts für Toxikologie, Bayer AG, Postfach 10 17 09, D-5600 Wuppertal 1, FRG

Lucchelli, P. E., M.D., Midy S.p.A., Sanofi Group, Via Piranesi, 38, I-20137 Milano, Italy

Mandahl, H., M.D., Deputy Director, Socialstyrelsen, The National Board of Health and Welfare, Department of Drugs, Box 607, S-751 25 Uppsala, Sweden

Marubini, E., Professor, M.D., Director of Istituto di Biometrica e Statistica Medica, Via G. Venezian 1, I-20133 Milano, Italy

Matsumura, A., M.D., Director, Biologics and Antibiotics Division, Pharmaceutical Affairs Bureau, Ministry of Health and Welfare, 2,2 1-Chome, Kasumigasaki, Chiyoda-ku, Tokyo 100, Japan

Miettinen, O. S., M.D., Ph.D., Professor of Epidemiology and Biostatistics, Prof. of Medicine, Faculty of Médicine, McGill University, 1020 Pine Avenue West, Montreal, Quebec H3A 1A2, Canada

Pejoviċ, M. H., Dept. of Med. Statistics, Institut G. Roussy, 94805 Villejuif, France

Poggiolini, D., Professor, M.D., General Director Pharmaceutical Division, Ministry of Health, Via della Civiltà Romana, 7, I-00144 Rome, Italy

Rawlins, M. D., M.D., Wolfson Unit of Pharmacology, The University, Newcastle-upon-Tyne NE1 7RU, Great Britain

Reinhardt, Prof. Dr. med., D., Universitäts-Kinderklinik, Moorenstrasse 5, D-4000 Düsseldorf, FRG

Schnieders, Prof. Dr. med., B., Direktor und Professor, Leiter des Instituts für Arneimittel des Bundesgesundheitsamtes, Seestrasse 10, D-1000 Berlin 65, FRG

Schwartz, D., Statistical Research Unit, National Institute of Health and Medical Research, 16 avenue Paul Vaillant Couturier, 94807 Villejuif Cedex, France

Sereni, F., Professor M.D., Chairman Department of Pediatrics, Clinica Pediatrica
Università, Via Commenda, 9, I-20122 Milano, Italy

Seyberth, Prof. Dr. med., H. W., Universitäts-Kinderklinik,
Im Neuenheimer Feld 150, D-6900 Heidelberg 1, FRG

Snell, E. S., MA MD FRCP, Director, Medical and Scientific Affairs, A.B.P.I.,
12 Whitehall, GB-London SW1A 2DY, Great Britain

Teijgeler, C. A., Dr. pharm., Chairman of the Committee for Proprietary Medicinal
Products, Doktor Reijersstraat 10, NL-2260 AK, Leideschendam, Netherlands

Vanderbeke, O., Dipl.-Math., Hoechst AG, Klinische Forschung,
Postfach 80 03 20, D-6230 Frankfurt 80, FRG

Walker, S. R., Professor, Centre for Medicines Research,
Carshalton Surrey SM5 4DS, Great Britain

Yaffe, S. J., M.D., Director, Center for Research for Mothers and Children,
National Institute of Child Health and Human Development,
National Institutes of Health, Building Landow, Room 7C03,
Bethesda, Maryland 20205, USA

Zbinden, Prof. Dr. med., G., Direktor, Institut für Toxikologie der Eidgenössischen
Technischen Hochschule und der Universität Zürich,
Schorenstrasse 16, CH-8603 Schwerzenbach bei Zürich, Switzerland

Zelen, M., Ph.D., Harvard School of Public Health,
677 Huntington Avenue, Boston, Mass. 02115, USA

Chronic toxicity tests, current problems and possible solutions

G. Zbinden

Conceptions and misconceptions

Chronic toxicity tests were originally designed to permit the detection and quantification of adverse properties of drugs and other chemicals to which humans are exposed for an extended period of time. Thus, the intention was not to study the acute toxic reactions, but rather the slowly developing lesions related to organ-directed toxicity, accumulation of the test substance or its metabolites in certain organs, functional and structural changes resulting from the continued necessity to metabolize and eliminate the foreign chemicals and to the gradual exhaustion of physiologic defense and repair mechanisms. The changes that one wanted to detect included adaptive processes such as cellular hypertrophy, proliferative reactions ranging from simple hyperplasia to benign and malignant tumors, metabolic disturbances such as fatty infiltration, glycogenosis and phospholipidosis, organ degenerations, e.g. atrophy, swelling and necrosis, and reactive responses such as inflammation, fibrosis and cirrhosis.

In order to reach these objectives with a reasonable effort and with the highest probability of not missing a relevant toxic effect, an omnibus procedure was devised that is characterized by the following features: 1) animals are exposed in the same manner as expected for humans, 2) to detect the adverse effects, clinical, biochemical and pathomorphological techniques used to diagnose human diseases are employed, 3) large numbers of laboratory animals of different species are included, and 4) the test substances are given at various dose levels, one of which must cause readily identifiable signs of toxicity.

Today, chronic toxicity tests are not only a regular, but the dominating and the most costly part of animal safety studies required before marketing of human and veterinary drugs, pesticides, consumer products, industrial chemicals and environmental pollutants. From this fact, one could conclude that the approach has stood the test of time and that its usefulness and necessity are generally acknowledged. That this is not the case is documented by the continuing debate about the predictive value of chronic toxicity tests and by cutting criticisms of regulatory safety requirements originating in the most diverse circles such as the pharmaceutical and chemical industry, the academic establishment and the antivivisectionist movement.

Understandably, the dissatisfaction with chronic toxicity tests is greatest among those who are concerned with the development of new drugs, particularly clinical pharmacologists and clinical investigators. That this is not a new phenomenon is documented by a statement made by a leading pharmacologist and toxicologist, John Barnes, thirty years ago. He wrote: "A chronic toxicity test is always a makeshift affair to be replaced as soon as possible by a more prominent structure of knowledge built on the foundations of physiology, biochemistry and other fundamental sciences" (Barnes and Denz 1954).

1

But despite his expectation that chronic toxicity tests would, in the near future, be replaced by something better, the procedures continue to be performed as before, and even the most modern regulatory guidelines, issued by national and international agencies, give no indication that the requirements for extensive chronic toxicity data would be lessened in the foreseeable future.

In this paper, the discussion will be limited to chronic toxicity testing of drugs for human use. The current problems in this important area can be traced to three main phenomena, namely: 1) misconceptions about the tests on the part of clinical pharmacologists and clinical investigators, 2) inherent imperfections of the animal models, and 3) inadequacies in designing and performing chronic toxicity tests.

Let us deal first with some of the misconceptions. Clinicians who review the preclinical safety data of new drugs are often appalled by the enormous volume of negative and seemingly irrelevant data that are provided by chronic toxicity tests. After having seen again and again such "data cemetries" that bear no resemblance to the responses observed in patients, they begin to doubt the scientific value and the logic behind the toxicologist's approach to safety evaluation. But clinicians rarely stop to think that no ethically acceptable alternative exists to this admittedly tedious and probably also wasteful procedure of assuring lack of unexpected organ toxicity, before a new drug can be administered to man. In addition, few clinicians ever hear of the many new substances that never reach the stage of human trials, because of adverse properties revealed in repeated-dose toxicity tests.

In other cases, clinical investigators are startled by the description of serious organ lesions caused intentionally and senselessly by overdosing rats and dogs in chronic toxicity studies. Although they may be aware that a certain amount of organ damage was intentionally induced by overdosing the animals, they are unable, based on the purely descriptive data provided, to judge the relevance for man. For this reason, the conclusion that such findings can be disregarded as experimental artifacts is quite often reached.

Another misconception of the clinicians is the belief that the toxicological information on new drugs is mainly contained in the section headed "toxicology" in the preclinical dossier. However, the repeated-dose toxicity studies that provide the bulk of the data contained in this section are only a small part of the information applicable to the safety of a new drug. Much additional evidence is found elsewhere, e.g. under the headings of pharmacology, endocrinology, drug disposition, even chemistry and physicochemistry.

From this discussion it is evident that the first problem regarding chronic toxicity testing of new drugs is mainly one of communication between the toxicologist who is using the experimental model, and the clinical investigator who must draw the relevant conclusions from the mass of data provided. The most important aspect in this dialogue is the clear understanding of the purpose of the chronic toxicity studies and the kind of lesions that are likely to be discovered by the procedure. From this, the clinician can then decide where some of the safety problems with a new drug may be expected. By being informed about the limitations of the experimental model, he will be able to decide where his responsibility for the patient's safety begins.

Inherent imperfections of the animal models

The major problems that plague the chronic toxicity testing of chemicals, are, as with most other animal models, those related to species differences. Surprisingly, little attention is paid to this matter in the course of routine development of drugs and other products. In order to illustrate this, let us consider one of the most important reasons for species differences, namely different pharmacokinetics and drug metabolism. Although many examples are known that demonstrate that poor predictability of toxic reactions in humans from animal experiments is due to differences in pharmacokinetics, drug metabolism or both, animal toxicity studies and biopharmaceutical investigations proceed quite independently from each other, both at their own pace, and very often at widely separated locations. A closer interaction between the two disciplines, experimental toxicology and biopharmaceutics, usually develops only if a "toxicological emergency" occurs. Some of such circumstances are listed in Table 1. In such cases, detailed biopharmaceutical investigations can often provide the data to permit a satisfactory solution of the toxicological problem. However, if no toxicological concern is created from the results of routine safety studies, biopharmaceutical data gathered in laboratory animals are, to a large extent, ignored. This is particularly the case with regard to the pharmacokinetic parameters. Normally, chronic toxicity tests are conducted according to standard protocols, whereby the test substances are given once daily by the route proposed to be used in humans. However, the elimination of the drug often proceeds at a much faster rate in the animals than in man. Thus, meaningful blood and tissue concentrations are maintained only for a short fraction of the day. As a consequence, the lack of toxicity in a chronic toxicity study may be entirely due to an inadequate dosing regimen. On the other hand, if the elimination half-life in the animals is long, daily administration of the compound may lead to drug accumulation and serious toxicity. But this toxic reaction may be quite irrelevant should such an accumulation not occur on therapeutic use of the drug in man.

From this discussion we can conclude that species differences concerning drug metabolism and pharmacokinetics represent one of the major problems for the interpretation of the results of chronic toxicity tests. However, if information about these variables were properly collected and available at the time when the toxicological studies are designed, chronic toxicity tests could be conducted in a much more realistic manner. Recognizing these facts, many pharmaceutical companies have begun to perform biopharmaceutical studies much earlier than before and to coordinate toxicological studies with biochemical investigations (Zbinden 1983). This effort requires an enormous investment in research facilities and scientific manpower. However, it will place the toxi-

Table 1. "Toxicological emergencies" calling for special collaborative efforts between toxicologists and biopharmaceutics.

1. Inability to satisfy protocol requirements (e.g. no toxic dose level achievable)
2. Positive findings in *in vitro* tests
3. Unusual and unexpected toxic response
4. Distinct species or sex differences, unexplained deaths
5. Doubts about acceptability of human trials
6. Accumulation of test compound, even in the absence of toxic reaction

cological investigations on a much more rational basis, will greatly improve the predictability of animal toxicity data, enhance the confidence in the preclinical safety evaluation and markedly reduce the inherent inadequacies of chronic toxicity tests.

Inadequacies in designing and performing chronic toxicity tests

In the introduction to this paper, the basic concepts of the chronic toxicity tests of chemicals were briefly characterized. In the last 40 years the experimental procedure has not changed significantly. Over the years, the quality of the laboratory animals has improved, the number of subjects included in the tests has increased, and the frequency and range of hematological and biochemical laboratory tests have been stepped up considerably. More organs are weighed at autopsy and more detailed histopathological examinations of the organs are performed. "Good Laboratory Practice" regulations have improved documentation, data processing and storage and the overall quality of the experimental procedures. But, as shown in Table 2, the data gathered from these extensive investigations still consist mainly of pathomorphological records and analytical determinations furnished by the clinical laboratory (Zbinden 1984).
In recent years the scope of toxicology has greatly expanded. In addition to the organ-directed lesions characterized by adaptive, proliferative, metabolic and reactive changes, many other undesirable consequences of chronic exposure to chemicals have been recognized. These include functional disturbances, e.g. of the cardiovascular, bronchopulmonary, gastrointestinal and nervous systems that can reach significant proportions without being associated with morphological alterations or biochemical aberrations (Zbinden 1984). Other areas of concern are behavioral disturbances, interference with the immune regulatory system, potential damage of repair mechanisms, acceleration of aging processes etc. It is evident that the standard protocol used for chronic toxicity studies is not capable of detecting many of these toxicologically rel-

Table 2. Data accumulated in a standard chronic toxicity study in rats (20 rats per dose and sex, 3 doses, 1 control).

Measurement	Frequency	Number of records
Body weight	Weekly	8 320
Food consumption	Weekly	4 166
General inspection	Daily	?
Clinical pathology (10 rats per dose and sex):		
Hematology (11 variables)	5×	4 400
Serum biochemistry (8 variables)	5×	3 200
Urine analysis (9 variables)	5×	3 600
Pathomorphology:		
Autopsy (all rats)		160
Organ weights (9 per rat)		1 440
Histopathology (36 organs, high dose and controls)		2 880
Total number of recorded determinations		28 646

4

evant responses. Therefore, great efforts must be made to widen the scope of toxicological investigations. Some progress is made in the area of functional measurements in chronic toxicity studies, mainly for the study of cardiovascular disturbances (Detweiler 1981, Zbinden 1981), and the discussion on means to investigate chronic damage of the immune regulatory system is well underway (Vos 1977, Falchetti et al. 1983).

In many other areas, however, chronic toxicity testing is still locked in a framework of traditional inflexibility. For example, a recent review of the laboratory procedures used to assess adverse effects on the hemostatic system has disclosed an almost total neglect of the pathophysiological research in this important field conducted in the past 20 years. Most toxicity studies we reviewed reported only platelet counts and repeated determinations of the prothrombin time, but these examinations were usually done in a large number of animals. Efforts to investigate all aspects of the hemostatic system, including plasmatic coagulation processes, platelet function and fibrinolysis, as is routine even in a modest clinical laboratory, are rarely if ever made in chronic toxicity tests. Likewise, the hazard of a thrombogenic effect is largely ignored by experimental toxicologists (Theus and Zbinden 1984). Other "areas of toxicological neglect" could also be cited, e.g. the problems of pulmonary function, social behavior and mental and motor performance.

While it is relatively easy to enumerate the methodological imperfections of current chronic toxicity testing and to complain about problems and inadequacies of the standard toxicological procedures, it is difficult to propose realistic solutions. It should also be noted that current methodology of chronic toxicity testing is highly standardized and under great constraint from regulatory agencies. Any deviation from the routine protocols is fraught with the danger of being accused of having disregarded current scientific standards. Moreover, test procedures to investigate many of the toxicological problems mentioned above are not yet developed, those that are proposed are mostly not properly validated and the relevance of their results is largely unknown. Thus, toxicologists in industry are reluctant to tread the risky path towards a new approach to the rapidly expanding problems of chronic toxicity.

Conclusions

Chronic toxicity testing as it is currently performed for drugs and many other chemicals has proven to be very useful for the detection of organ-directed toxicity that manifests itself by pathomorphological lesions of the organs and aberrations of biochemical determinations in body fluids. It is difficult to estimate how many human lives have been saved and how much suffering has been averted thanks to the early detection of hazardous chemicals in routine chronic toxicity tests. However, I am convinced that the number of dangerous substances that were recognized and consequently prevented from entering the human environment is considerable. Thus, chronic toxicity testing of drugs and other products, despite the acknowledged shortcomings of the procedures, cannot be abandoned now or in the foreseeable future.

Criticisms of the chronic toxicity tests by clinical pharmacologists and clinical investigators are, in part, due to unrealistic expectations. The experimental design of the procedure is such that a limited number of toxic responses are detected, and many toxic responses occurring in humans, e.g. anaphylactic and allergic reactions, just cannot be demonstrated with the chronic toxicity model. In addition, toxicological methodology always incorporates a "worst case design" by intentionally producing toxicity through overdosing. With this approach, the toxicologist wishes to learn about the adverse properties of the chemical per se (hazard detection) without any concern for the eventual determination of human risk under realistic exposure conditions. Organ damage detected under such circumstances creates great problems for the clinical investigator, as it provides little information about the danger of the drug for research subjects, but puts him in an awkward position with regard to the patients who have the right to full disclosure of preclinical data, and ethical review boards that mainly consist of individuals even less qualified to assess the significance of the experimental findings.

An even greater problem is the inadequacy of the animal model and the difficulties of extrapolating findings in chronic toxicity tests to man. In this area progress is being made by a more systematic incorporation of biopharmaceutical investigations into the design of toxicological experiments. This is particularly true for the pharmacokinetic investigations which facilitate the development of dosing regimens that result in exposure levels of the laboratory animals more akin to those ocurring in man.

Finally, it is stressed that the methodology of chronic toxicity testing is in great need of a critical review. Research in physiology and on pathophysiological mechanisms of many diseases have pointed to a large number of targets for toxicological action that are not considered in chronic toxicity testing. Methods are, therefore, under development which permit the detection of functional disturbances of many organ systems. Much research is still needed to develop adequate experimental models and to validate them with appropriate reference substances. This will ultimately result in a scientific and quantitative assessment of a large variety of potential toxicological characteristics of the test compounds. With this approach, more meaningful safety data will be generated, and confidence in the scientific value of chronic toxicity tests will be restored.

References

1. Barnes JM, Denz FA (1954) Experimental methods used in determining chronic toxicity. Pharmacol Rev 6:191–242
2. Detweiler DK (1981) The use of electrocardiography in toxicological studies with beagle dogs. In: Balazs T (ed) Cardiac Toxicology, Vol III, CRC Press Inc, Boca Raton, Fla, p 33–82
3. Falchetti R, Silvestri S, Battaglia A, Caprino L (1983) Toxicological evaluation of immunomodulating drugs. In: Zbinden G, Cohadon F, Detaille JY, Mazué G (eds) Current Problems in Drug Toxicology. John Libbey Eurotext, Paris, London, p 248–263
4. Theus R, Zbinden G (1984) Toxicological assessment of the hemostatic system, regulatory requirements and industry practice. Regulatory Toxicol Pharmacol 4:74–95
5. Vos JG (1977) Immune suppression as related to toxicology. Crit Rev Toxicol 5:67–101
6. Zbinden G (1981) Assessment of cardiotoxic effects in subacute and chronic rat toxicity studies. In: Balazs T (ed) Cardiac Toxicity, Vol III. CRC Press Inc, Boca Raton, Fla, p 7–32
7. Zbinden G (1983) Metabolic studies in chemical safety evaluation. In: Caldwell J, Paulsen GD (eds) Foreign Compound Metabolism. Taylor and Francis Ltd, London, p 203–211
8. Zbinden G (1984) Neglect of function and obsession with structure in toxicity testing. Proceedings, 9th International Congress of Pharmacology, London, Vol 1, p 43–49

Author's address:
Prof. Dr. med. G. Zbinden
Institute of Toxicology,
Swiss Federal Institute of Technology
University of Zürich
Schorenstraße 16
CH-8603 Schwerzenbach
Switzerland

What can be gained from a retrospective analysis of chronic toxicity studies?

Stuart R. Walker

Introduction

Animal testing for pharmaceutical compounds is of value in defining their toxicity and assessing the predicted safety of their use in man. Recently there has been increasing pressure to produce "safer" drugs; the implication often being to carry out a more extensive safety evaluation programme. In contrast, there is increasing pressure to rationalise and where possible to decrease the amount of animal toxicology required in connection with the process of drug development. Any prospect, however, of achieving a balance between increased reliance on the predictive value of animal studies and the rational use of animal resources must stem from a re-appraisal of conventional animal testing procedures, and improved experimental design based on the better use of available toxicological data of previously investigated compounds.

Regulations

National regulatory authorities differ in their guidelines for appropriate safety evaluation studies with new drugs and this has an impact on the animal investigations carried out by pharmaceutical companies in order to satisfy licencing requirements. These have in many cases proliferated over the past twenty years and it is now important to have some method for assessing the value of the animal studies specified. The most expensive, time consuming and controversial animal toxicology study is the long-term or chronic study (Heywood 1983). In order to obtain marketing approval for a medicine which is to be administered clinically for six months or longer the recommended duration of animal exposure in two species (one rodent and one non-rodent) ranges from six months for EEC countries, to twelve months for the United States and eighteen months for the Canadian authorities (Table 1). These differences are surprising as presumably

Table 1. Recommendations for the minimum duration of animal toxicity studies

Proposed duration of human exposure	Duration of animal toxicity studies required for product licence application		
	Canada	EEC	USA
Up to 1 week	4–6 m	4 w	up to 3 m
Up to 1 month	18 m	3 m	up to 6 m
Up to 3 months	18 m	6 m	up to 6 m
6 months – unlimited	18 m	6 m	12 m (non-r)
			18 m (r)

the rationale that leads to different toxicity testing requirements is based on the same sets of data generated and provided to the Regulatory Authorities by the Pharmaceutical Industry. There is increasing concern about chronic toxicity studies in view of the claims that studies of longer than a few weeks are rarely necessary to predict unwanted side effects. Therefore, an appreciation of both the limitations of animal data and the potential value of retrospective analyses of such toxicological data has led to a major research initiative in the establishment of a toxicology databank for pharmaceutical compounds.

Toxicology databank

Despite many critisms toxicological investigations in living animals are currently the best method available for predicting potential human hazards, and these pre-clinical safety evaluation studies provide the basis for carrying out clinical research ethically and "safely". However, there is little published information on the additional value, if any, of long-term animal toxicology studies compared with short-term studies (less than six months) in predicting adverse effects for man; and the rationale for these studies must therefore be questioned. One approach to determining their value is to carry out a retrospective analysis of the data generated by pharmaceutical companies to satisfy regulatory requirements. However, to date these data have been confined to the archives of the companies and Regulatory Authorities and the problems of confidentiality, time and resources have not permitted their evaluation. These difficulties have now been overcome and a number of pharmaceutical companies in Europe have released such data.

Thirteen pharmaceutical companies with research and development activities directed from the U.K. have provided comprehensive repeated dose toxicology data for compounds tested and evaluated since 1965, and these data have been used to establish a computer based toxicology databank. Companies were asked to select those compounds for which data from chronic toxicity studies were available which would allow a comparison between short (less than six months) and long-term (more than six months) animal studies. Carcinogenicity studies were not included unless a combined carcinogenicity/toxicity study had been carried out. A detailed questionnaire was used to collect these data, which included details of chemical and therapeutic class, the animal species investigated, the route of administration, elimination half-life, LD_{50} in the species under investigation, dose levels utilised, number of animals included in each dose group and the duration of the study. Further information required included clinical signs relating to various body systems, laboratory findings (haematology, clinical chemistry and urinalysis) and salient pathological changes where these were thought to be drug related. All data were entered onto a Sirius Microcomputer using "Delta", a commercial software programme from Compsoft (Lumley & Walker 1984). This is a dynamic programme that stores information in multi-level files divided into records and sub-divided into fields and allows comprehensive analysis of the data. The header record contains a great deal of important background data (Fig. 1), and a transaction group (several fields automatically repeated) was used to enter all effects when these first and subsequently occurred, and the dose and number of animals affected.

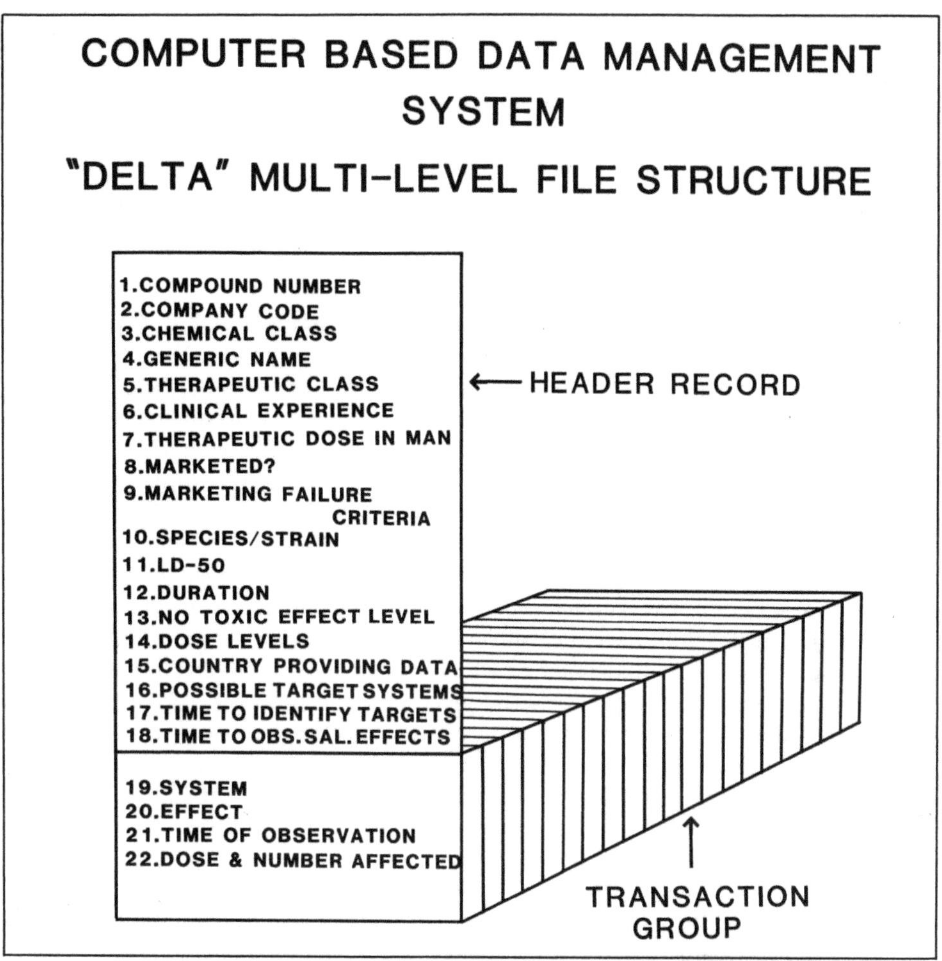

Fig. 1. Computer-based data management system – "Delta" multi-level file structure.

Analysis of animal toxicology

Comprehensive toxicological data for seventy-four pharmaceutical compounds were provided by the thirteen pharmaceutical companies approached in the United Kingdom. For fifty of these compounds extensive clinical data is available and fifty-eight of the compounds have been studied in more than one species. Major therapeutic categories represented include gastrointestinal drugs, cardiovascular drugs and diuretics, respiratory system drugs, central nervous system drugs, anti-infective agents and anti-allergic compounds. These seventy-four compounds resulted in one hundred and forty-five case studies, where a case study is defined as one compound administered to one species by the same route for one or more time periods and including several dose levels for each test period. Of the one hundred and forty-five case studies, in ninety-three the maximum period of animal exposure was six months or less while in fifty-two the maximum duration of treatment was twelve, eighteen or twenty-four months. Of these fifty-two case studies, twenty-two were in the rat, eighteen in the dog and twelve in primates.

A comparative analysis of short- and long-term toxicity studies has been carried out in order to determine what new information, if any, is to be gained from studies of longer than six months. In forty-five out of the fifty-two case studies available for analysis both short- and long-term tests had been carried out. These forty-five case studies involve thirty-two compounds of which seventeen were not marketed for clinical, commercial or toxicological reasons, but not due to any new information uncovered after 6 months study.

In all forty-five case studies the target organs were identified within six months. In twenty of these, all toxicological effects were seen within six months. No six month data are available in nine of the remaining twenty-five case studies, so although apparently new effects were seen in the long-term studies, no conclusions can be drawn as to whether these effects would have been apparent by six months with a different study design. It is relevant that for time and dose dependent effects, in six of these nine cases, the same or higher doses were used in the long-term compared with the short-term study. In a further seven case studies all the findings after six months were not considered to be completely new effects, but extensions of those observed in the short-term investigations. In three case studies, the findings after six months were considered to be of no toxicological significance, i.e., shivering and colouration of gut contents. In two out of the twenty-five case studies, the new findings had been seen in an alternative species within six months (liver weight increase; glycosuria and urinary casts). Again in both these case studies, the same or higher doses were used in the long-term study. In the remaining four cases, the new effects seen after six months did not influence the development of the compounds and their progression to market or termination of their research. Again in three of these latter cases, the same or higher doses were used in the long-term compared to the short-term study.

It appears therefore that study design, including dose levels used, the number of animals employed and the parameters measured, is a major factor in determining whether or not salient toxicological effects are observed within six months.

Discussion

Previous attempts (Bein 1963, Peck 1968, McNamara 1976) to determine the value of long-term animal studies have concluded that there is little, if any, new information to be gained from investigations beyond three to six months. In this retrospective analysis, target organs were identified in all case studies within one, three or six months. Whilst apparently new effects were identified in some case studies after six months, either these were extensions of the effects seen within six months, the same effects had been observed in the alternative species within 6 months, or the effects were not of sufficient toxicological significance to affect the subsequent development of the compound. These data do not therefore support the need for animal toxicity studies of longer than six months duration apart from those designed to investigate carcinogenicity.

In addition to the results described in this paper, data on repeated dose animal studies of varying duration are available to the Centre for Medicines Research from pharmaceutical companies in Switzerland, Germany and the United States. When this information has been verified and the data are compatible with the U.K. database, they will be included in future analyses. The establishment of this computer-based toxicology databank is a major initiative towards determining the value of animal data obtained during longer term studies and exploring the discrepancies between the regulatory requirements of different countries.

References

1. Bein HD (1963) Rational and Irrational Numbers in Toxicology. Proc Eur Soc Study Drug Tox 2:15–24
2. Heywood R (1983) Long-Term Toxicity. Animals and Alternatives in Toxicity Testing. Proceedings of a meeting held at the Royal Society of London, Nov 1982. Balls M, Riddell RJ, Worden AN (eds). Academic Press, London 1983:171–179
3. Lumley CE and Walker SR (1984) The Establishment of a Computer-Based Toxicology Databank. Medical Informatics. In Press
4. McNamara BP (1976) Concepts in Health Evaluation of Commercial and Industrial Chemicals. In: New Concepts in Safety Evaluation. Mehlman, Shapiro and Blumenthal (eds). Wiley, New York 1976:61–115
5. Peck HM (1968) An Appraisal of Drug Safety Evaluation in Animals and the Extrapolation of Results to Man. In: Importance of Fundamental Principles in Drug Evaluation. Tedeschi and Tedeschi (eds). Raven Press 1968:449–471

Author's address:
Professor Stuart R. Walker
Centre for medicines research
Carshalton
Surrey SM5 4DS
U.K.

The role of carcinogenicity studies in risk assessment

E. Fröhlich and R. Hess

Introduction

Until recently, most of the controversy about carcinogenicity testing and long-term safety has been concerned with food additives and environmental chemicals rather than with drugs. However, in medicine, cytotoxic drugs or photochemotherapy are used with increasing frequency for the treatment of non-malignant disorders. The occurrence of malignancy in spontaneous or induced immunodeficiency disease has also become a more frequent finding. This has opened the view to possible long-term consequences of certain forms of chemotherapy. Furthermore, for drugs in general which are intended for longer-term use, the question of carcinogenicity has become, from the regulatory point of view, most decisive for the fate of a new product.

The need to investigate the carcinogenic potential of a drug was confirmed a year ago by the EEC Council by amending its 1975 directive (EEC 1983). Carcinogenicity testing shall normally be required for substances likely to be administrated regularly over a prolonged period of a patient's life, for substances having close chemical analogy with known carcinogenic or cocarcinogenic compounds, for substances which have given rise to suspicious results during long-term toxicological tests, or in tests designed to reveal mutagenicity, or in other short-term carcinogenicity tests.

The value of short-term tests

There is ample evidence that DNA damage brought about by reactive compounds or electrophilic intermediates, and expressed as mutations, DNA repair or cell transformation, is involved in the induction of cancer. During the last two decades a new area of research has grown from genetics which has led to a revolution in the methods of toxicological evaluation (De Serres 1976). New methodology has evolved to determine genotoxins, denoting those mutagens which interact with the genetic material and which are capable of inducing point mutations, chromosome aberrations or genome mutations. In order to identify potential mutagens with reasonable certainty, a number of suitable *in vitro* and *in vivo* models have been developed. It is indispensable to apply models which are capable of detecting the various forms of mutations, for it is impossible to extrapolate from one mutation to another. Results derived from experiments on submammalian or *in vitro* systems are usually considered to be of limited predictive value with regard to possible effects on the human genome. However, they are highly sensitive and serve as early indicators for genetic damage. The most commonly used test is the Salmonella typhimurium reversion assay developed by Ames and coworkers (Ames et al. 1975, McCann et al. 1975). Because of the essentially nonquantitative conditions inherent in the Ames protocol and because of the incompleteness of its metabolic activation system, the results of the test cannot be used directly for extrapolation, i.e. for the prediction of human risk. Nevertheless, of 30 human carcinogens which have been evaluated by the International Agency or Research on Cancer, 70% were detected as mutagens (Bartsch and Tomatis 1983). Other comparisons with suspected carcinogens suggest that with the use of the Ames test more than 80% may be identified today as mutagens (McCann et al. 1975). However, there are a number of agents which are definitely carcinogenic and which are not readily detectable as mutagens, e.g. sex hormones.

The new EEC directive recommends the systematic application of short-term mutagenicity and carcinogenicity tests but concludes that the only practical approach for assessing the carcinogenic activity of drugs is the performance of formal long-term studies in rodents. Confidence in positive carcinogenicity test results is increased when they are confirmed in multiple short-term tests using non-repetitive endpoints and different activation systems (Bartsch and Tomatis 1983).

Regarding the use of short-term tests in risk assessment, the problem is a matter of establishing a quantitative relationship between the potency of a carcinogen in experimental animals and its genotoxic activity in appropriate tests. Correlations which could be used in the assessment of risk of chemicals are usually of a highly complex nature, and rather inconsistent patterns are expected when larger numbers and different types of chemicals are compared. Thus, the analysis of 465 compounds with known or suspected carcinogenic activity has yielded unsatisfactorily low correlations for some categories of chemicals (Rinkus and Legator 1979). On the other hand, certain chemicals such as monofunctional alkylating agents provide rather consistent patterns of mutagenic response and carcinogenic activity. In this way, the "specific mutagenicity" may be calculated which differs within six orders of magnitude (McCann et al. 1975). Similarly large differences are demonstrated when a comparison is drawn between the mutagenic and the carcinogenic potency of a selected series of substances (Meselson and Russell 1977).

Both positive and negative data from short-term tests are used in setting priorities for carcinogenicity studies but they do not by themselves provide the basis for risk assessment. This is mainly due to the limitations of even an extensive battery of tests to detect all possible stages involved in carcinogenesis and because of the uncertainty as to which mechanism is operative for a particular chemical or metabolite.

Relevance and limitations of long-term studies in rodents

Provided that sufficient data are available for valid comparison, a good qualitative correlation is usually observed between carcinogenic effects in man and carcinogenic effects in experimental animals (IARC 1982). This indicates that findings obtained in long-term carcinogenicity studies in rodents may be of value in predicting a similar effect in man. This does not imply, however, that all experimental carcinogens will be active in man. It should be stressed that epidemiological studies have strong limitations in sensitivity. Therefore, the position is taken that positive results from well conducted animal studies provide strong evidence of carcinogenic hazard in man (NTP 1984).

14

Extrapolations from rodents to man for preventive purposes always represent best estimates rather than scientifically validated data. For this reason, the term "sufficient" or "limited" evidence of carcinogenicity, used by IARC (IARC 1982) for classification purposes, refers only to the evidence available and not to the potency of the carcinogenic effect, nor to the mechanism involved.

The evaluation and interpretation of long-term studies involves several important methodological aspects. A typical example of a carcinogenicity study in laboratory rodents is an experiment with a total number of 900 rats, of which on an average 40 different tissues will be examined microscopically, will produce 10,000 to 25,000 histopathological diagnoses. This body of data is to be analysed and to be correlated to the individual survival times of the animals to reveal evidence for treatment related production of tumours. A "tumourigenic activity" of a compound may be assumed when statistical evidence indicating a higher probability for tumour occurrence in treated animals than in untreated controls results from the analysis.

The effect under investigation (i.e. the incidence of animals bearing a specific tumour) is masked and confounded by conditions which are either unknown to the investigator or which are outside his control. This situation leads easily to the misinterpretation of the results. Only a "good" experiment may truly reveal the compound-related effects. The requirements for a "good" experiment (Table 1) were compiled by D.R. Cox as early as 1958 (Cox 1958).

When the treatment (compound and exposure route), the experimental units (species and number of animals) and the nature of observation (histopathological criteria) have been decided upon, the design and the conduct of a chronic study must be envisaged to meet these requirements as closely as possible in order to obtain the desired information on possible carcinogenicity. A few examples may illustrate principal problems which influence the value of such a study.

The *absence of systematic error* is the first requirement to be fulfilled when planning, conducting and evaluating an experiment. Randomisation is a necessary but not sufficient condition to achieve the absence of systematic error in long-term studies. Following randomisation, untreated control animals receiving the normal diet should not differ from those being exposed to the bioactive compound in their diet. The protection offered by randomisation against systematic error is however not complete. Due to the large size of a typical long-term study, and due to the particular nature of histopathological evaluation, there are additional sources of systematic errors. Among these are the differences between observers (e.g. when several pathologists are involved in the diagnostic work), or time-dependent shifts of diagnostic criteria (when one pathologist

Table 1. Requirements for a good experiment

---

1. Absence of systematic error
2. Precision
3. Range of validity
4. Simplicity
5. Calculation of uncertainty

Table 2. Precision of an experiment

---

1. Intrinsic variability of the experimental material
2. The accuracy of the experimental work
3. The number of experimental units
4. The number of repeat observations per experimental unit
5. The design of the experiment
6. The method of analysis

---

performs the diagnostic work during a longer period). Special measures are necessary to reduce the occurrence of this type of systematic error. Thus, long-term studies have a greater inclination to be affected by systematic errors than tests of short duration and smaller size.

The *precision of an experiment* is another requirement to be fulfilled. It is influenced by a number of well-known factors (Table 2). For practical purposes, a long-term study consisting of 500–1000 animals represents the upper limit of practical feasibility. Assuming that 5 dose-groups per sex are appropriate, the carcinogenicity screening will be limited to dose-groups containing 50–100 animals. The limitation of resolution results directly from this small number of experimental units (Fleiss 1973) which often demonstrate a high intrinsic variability of the parameters under study. Furthermore, statistical intergroup comparisons do not permit determination of threshold values. The direct derivation of so-called safe doses is therefore not possible. Neither does the "megamouse" approach resolve these problems (Hughes et al. 1983), even by using 24,000 animals as in the ED01 study (Staffa and Mehlman 1980). Statistical problems make it impossible to prove or to disprove the existence of thresholds (Hess et al. 1981), or, in the face of marked effects at the high exposure levels, to discriminate between lack of significant effect and lack of a real treatment-related effect at low exposure level (Mantel 1984). Thus, with regard to its objectives, the chronic carcinogenicity study is an experiment of limited precision.

The *range of validity* of long-term studies is ill-defined. The selection of doses for a carcinogenicity study is based on the concept of maximum tolerated dose (MTD). Observations made near an MTD may not be relevant to conditions of actual human exposure because the biological mechanisms working in the range of actual human exposure may be quite different from those working at exposure ranges similar to the MTD (Rodricks and Taylor 1983, Ciminera et al. 1984).

Simplicity of experimental design is mandatory to avoid responses which are too complex. Usually, this requirement is fulfilled in long-term studies. The simplicity of design in toxicological studies does however sharply contrast with the sometimes complex interdependence of different types of lesions under investigation (Salsburg 1980). It is well known that the effects of a treatment on longevity and on tumour occurrence have to be carefully disentangled when evaluating a long-term study (Peto et al. 1980, Gart et al. 1979).

The data produced by an experiment should permit the *calculation of the uncertainty*, i.e. the standard error for the intergroup differences from which the limits of error for

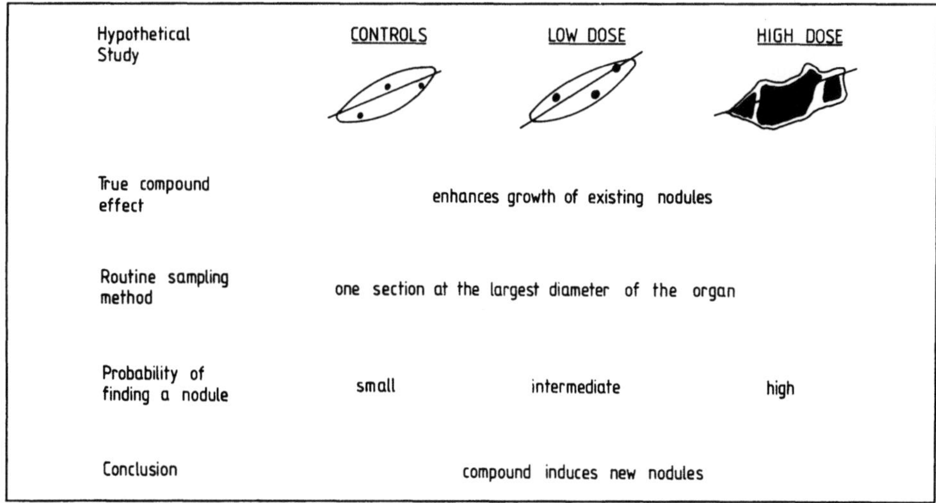

Fig. 1. Sampling error (tumour occurrence).

the true difference can be calculated at the required level of probability. A necessary prerequisite is the good quality of the histopathological data which should avoid major errors, e.g. in sampling (Fig. 1).

Conclusion

Evidence is increasing that carcinogenesis proceeds through a multistep process described as initiation, promotion and progression (Weinstein et al. 1984). A chemical carcinogen may affect each of these stages by various mechanisms. Initiation, for instance, results from heritable (mutational) changes in DNA of susceptible somatic cells. The multistep hypothesis of cancer development is expected ultimately to provide the scientific tools for a realistic assessment of human risk. At present, however, we must rely on animal experiments which suffer from shortcomings of different sources, but which, despite their limitations, offer the criteria of a broad classification for carcinogenic potential (IARC 1902), or for potency on qualitative and quantitative grounds (Theiss 1983).

Ultimately, carcinogenicity studies in animals generate hypotheses for further specific experimental investigation of pathogenetic mechanisms. In the case of non-genotoxic compounds for instance, which enhance liver-cell tumour formation in rodents, a promotion study may demonstrate the mechanism underlying hepatocarcinogenesis (Farber 1982).

The results of long-term carcinogenicity studies may be used to fit statistical or stochastic models of tumor incidences as a function of the dose and possibly also of other parameters (such as time-to-tumour). By this means, "Virtually safe doses" may be estimated which may form the rationale for quantitative risk assessment (Food Safety Council 1980).

Our knowledge of the biological events in the presumed multistep or multi-stage process leading to the formation of tumours is still limited. The long-term study, however, is the only means which may demonstrate unequivocally the full expression of compound-related tumourigenesis. The value of the long-term study depends crucially on additional experiments investigating mechanisms which may be involved in the pathogenesis of the compound-related tumours. The multidisciplinary approach presently used in experimental carcinogenesis can be expected to provide critical data for the quantitative and qualitative assessment of risk to the patient so as to balance it against the benefit which is derived from a particular treatment.

References

1. Ames BN, McCann J, Yamasaki E (1975) Methods for Detecting Carcinogens and Mutagens with the Salmonella/mammalian-microsome mutagenicity test. Mutat Res 31:347–364
2. Bartsch H, Tomatis L (1983) Comparison between Carcinogenicity and Mutagenicity Based on Chemicals Evaluated in the IARC Monographs. Environ Health Perspec 47:305–317
3. Ciminera JL, Heyse JF, Mantel N, Pitot HC (1984) Design of Cancer Assays for Pharmaceutical Agents. Letter to the Editor. Nat Cancer Inst 72:1212
4. Cox DR (1958) Planning of Experiments. Wiley, New York (Probability and Statistic Series)
5. DeSerres (1976) Prospects for a Revolution in the Methods of Toxicological Evaluation. Mutat Res 38:165–176
6. EEC (1983) Council Directive of 26 October 1983 amending Directives 65/65/EEC, 75/318/EEC and 75/319/EEC on the Approximations of Provisions laid down by law, regulation or administration action relating to proprietary medicinal products (83/570/EEC). Off J Eur Commun L332/1-10
7. Farber E (1982) Chemical carcinogenesis, a biological perspective. Am J Pathol 106:271–296
8. Fleiss JL (1973) Statistical Methods for Rates and Proportions. Wiley Series in probability and mathematical statistics. Wiley, New York
9. Food Safety Council (1980). Quantitative Risk Assessment. Food Cosmet. Toxicol 18:711–734
10. Gart JJ, Chu KC, Tarone RE (1979) Statistical Issues in Interpretation of Chronic Bioassay Tests for Carcinogenicity. J Nat Cancer Inst 62:957–974
11. Hess R, Waechter F, Bentley P (1981) Zur Thematik des experimentellen Schwellenwertes in der Karzinogenese. AMI-Berichte 2:219–226
12. Hughes DH, Bruce RD, Hart RW, Fishbein L, Gaylor DW, Carlton WW (1983) A Report on the Workshop on Biological and Statistical Implications of the ED01 Study and Related Data Bases. Fund Appl Toxicol 3:129–136
13. IARC (1982) IARC Monographs on the Evaluation of the Carcinogenic Risk of Chemicals to Humans. Supplement 4, Chemicals, Industrial Processes and Industries Associated with Cancer in humans. IARC Monographs, Volumes 1 to 29. International Agency for Research on Cancer, Lyon
14. Mantel N (1984) Treatment of Interim Deaths and Low Dose Responses in Bioassay. Letter to the Editor. Risk Analysis 4:81–82
15. McCann J, Choi E, Yamasaki E (1975) Detection of Carcinogens as Mutagens in the Salmonella/Microsome Test: Assay of 300 Chemicals. Proc Natl Acad Sci USA 72:5135–5139
16. McCann J, Ames BN (1977) The Salmonella/Microsome Mutagenicity Test: Predictive Value for Animal Carcinogenicity. In: Hiatt HH, Watson JD, Winsten JA (eds) Origins of Human Cancer. Cold Spring Harbor Laboratory, New York, pp 1431–1450
17. Meselson M, Russell K (1977) Comparison of Carcinogenic and Mutagenic Potency. In: Hiatt HH, Watson JD, Winsten JA (eds) Origins of Human Cancer. Cold Spring Harbor Laboratory, New York, pp 1473–1481
18. NTP (1984) Report of the Ad Hoc Panel on Chemical Carcinogenesis Testing and evaluation of the National Toxicology Program. Board of Scientific Counselors, August 17, 1984

19. Peto R, Pike MC, Day NE, Gray RG, Lee PN, Parish S, Peto J, Richards S, Wahrendorf J (1980) Guidelines for Simple, Sensitive Significance Tests for Carcinogenic Effects in Long-term Animal Experiments (Annex). In: Long-Term and Short-Term Screening Assays for Carcinogens: A Critical Appraisal. IARC Monographs, Supplement 2. International Agency for Research on Cancer. Lyon, p 311 425
20. Rinkus SJ, Legator MS (1979) Chemical Characterization of 465 Known or Suspected Carcinogens and Their Correlation with Mutagenic Activity in the Salmonella typhimurium system. Cancer Res 39:3289–3318
21. Rodricks J, Taylor MR (1983) Application of Risk Assessment to Food Safety Decision Making. Regulat Toxicol Pharmacol 3:275–307
22. Salsburg D (1980) The Effects of Lifetime Feeding Studies on Patterns of Senile Lesions in Mice and Rats. Drug Chem Toxicol 3:1–33
23. Staffa JA, Mehlman MA (1980) Innovations in Cancer Risk Assessment (ED01 Study). J Environ Pathol Toxicol (Special Issue) 3:1–246
24. Theiss JC (1983) The Ranking of Chemicals for Carcinogenic Potency. Regulat Toxicol Pharmacol 3:220–328
25. Weinstein IB, Gattoni-Celli S, Kirschmeyer P, Lambert M, Hsiao W, Backer J, Jeffrey A (1984) Molecular Mechanisms in Multistage Chemical Carcinogenesis. In: Greim H, Jung R, Kramer M, Marquardt H (eds) Biochemical Basis of Chemical Carcinogenesis, 13th Workshop Conference HOECHST. Raven Press, New York, pp 193–212

Authors' address:
Dr. med. E. Fröhlich
Toxicology
Ciba-Geigy
CH-4002 Basel
Switzerland

Alternatives to chronic toxicity studies

Rolf Baß, Peter Grosdanoff, Toni Lehnert

Introduction

Testing for chronic toxicity plays an important role in the overall evaluation of the toxic potential of chemical substances. It is routinely performed *in vivo*, i.e. in whole rodent and nonrodent animals. Certain rules and regulations exist that govern the form of performance of chronic toxicity testing for different sectors of our chemical world, for example, OECD regulations for testing of chemicals, EEC and FDA regulations for testing pharmaceutical substances. The requirements differ in regard to the number and selection of species, number of animals per dose group and experiment, modes of application and duration of experiment.
The topic chosen for this contribution raises expectations that are hard to meet.
During the last few years our attention has been focused more and more on this type of toxicological investigation which somehow builds the center for understanding untoward drug effects. It has been in this demanding position for quite some time now, although groups holding different interests and attitudes have tried to give it different shapes. Attempts to update chronic toxicity testing have been governed, guided and bound by scientific ability, industrial standards, governmental regulations and consumer expectations. This explains why changes for the better are very seldom.

Present-day chronic toxicity studies

What type of information do we expect from chronic toxicity studies today? What do we want to detect? We *have* to detect an enormous number of facts, details and connections, especially organ changes and changes in the *function* of organs and systems, their acting together, in sequence and interdependence. The connections and the interdependence of heart and vascular function, kidneys, lung, CNS, and hormonal influences, for example, are most obvious. When accepting this goal, we also have to accept the fact that chronic toxicity studies cannot be replaced by some *in vitro* experiments or cell cultures. In consequence, we have to state that chronic toxicity studies can only be replaced by chronic toxicity studies. This does not imply, however, that chronic toxicity studies have not changed or will not change. We have come to realize that rather than using a shotgun approach to make the black box unravel its contents of possible toxic events, it is more advisable to apply fine tools – analytical, pathological and clinical ones – for their detection and understanding.

Notes for guidance of EEC and other regulations

Requirements and means to perform repeated dose toxicity studies in EEC countries have recently been published (1). Chronic toxicity studies can be of a preliminary type,

Table 1. Duration of chronic toxicity studies

Type: preliminary, routine
Duration: related to intended duration of treatment

Clinical	Pre-clinical
1 day	2 weeks (4 weeks)
7 days	4 weeks (3 months)
30 days	3 months (4 weeks, 6 months)
beyond	6 months (3 months, 12 months)

routine type, or of a third type which deals with the investigation of special problems. During the last few years we Europeans have changed our attitude to this classification. However, there is still a clear-cut correlation between the intended duration of treatment in man and the duration of pre-clinical chronic toxicity studies (Table 1). As a first alternative to classical concepts of chronic toxicity studies, which lasted for up to 18 or even 24 months, duration of animal chronic toxicity studies now, as a rule, only last up to 6 months. These 6-month animal studies apply to unlimited clinical trials and use in man; for shorter clinical studies and use, they have been adjusted accordingly. Some other countries still insist on longer animal studies (e.g. Japan, USA, Canada). We Europeans expect that the duration of chronic toxicity studies for more than 6 months can be replaced by the very high systemic exposure to high doses. In some cases a high – toxic – dosage that can be applied for 6 months must be reduced for longer studies. As a result, some toxicity might be overlooked. This may be due to adaptation processes, as is known e.g. for intermittent increase in glucose levels returning to normal later on.

All cases claiming to depict in toxicity some organ or other only after 12 or 18 months of treatment are likely to be detected either earlier or by some special investigations. This represents the second alternative to conventional chronic toxicity testing: replacement of chronic toxicity studies lasting for more than 6 months by including special investigations uncovering toxic signs, for example, in the eye, ear, kidney, pancreas, and liver. Methods to make high doses reach such organs or to induce neurotoxicity are available. For the time being and for understandable reasons exemptions exist where testing for more than 6 months and using lower doses appears feasible, i.e. nonsteroidal antiphlogistics. Ulcerations induced by high doses might inhibit the development of other types of toxicity. Unspecific reactions or excessive pharmacological actions of high doses may mask specific toxic reactions. Sleep for almost 24 hrs a day may be a sign of toxicity but not necessarily the one sought. This explains the difficulties which sometimes arise in planning and performing the right experiment, the choice of dose levels, dosing intervals, or duration of treatment. A rule allowing experimentation on a shorter level (i.e., less than 6 months) must then be broken.

Preliminary information on chronic toxicity is needed for planning further studies, be it for more chronic studies, be it for carcinogenicity studies. We have come across a well-publicized case where a very reactive chemical substance was not adequately tested by such range finding for carcinogenicity studies. The carcinogenicity study performed yielded nasal tumors with high incidence at the highest dose tested. But many animals had died at an early stage without having developed tumors due to the toxicity of the chemical.

Although good laboratory practice is meant to prevent such an outcome of a study, it clearly shows the necessity of preliminary studies, for example, to uncover the steepness of the dose-response curve and the occurrence of toxic indications (Table 2). Range finding is also useful for planning reproduction toxicity studies. However, we have to keep in mind that doses toxic to the pregnant female can differ from those toxic to non-pregnant animals.

Mutagenicity studies are often planned and based on LD50 values, sometimes obtained in different laboratories and by using different strains of animals. Instead of doing so we should think about range finding for such mutagenicity studies by employing data from preliminary chronic toxicity studies. These examples show *where* preliminary chronic toxicity studies can be used to obtain additional information for *other* toxicological studies.

Similarly, data obtained from chronic toxicity studies can be used to check on data from pharmacological animal experiments, usually done for short periods only. Routine chronic toxicity studies are to reveal target organ toxicity, interactions between organs, functions and systems. This may sometimes include preliminary information on the tumor-inducing capability of the drug. Altogether the aim is to detect morbidity rather than mortality (Table 3).

The next change to be introduced into classical chronic toxicity testing concerns species selection and number of animals used. In the EEC, as a rule, the number of experimental species has already been decreased to two, one usually being a non-rodent. Along the lines of obtaining other pertinent information *earlier* than we are still used to, it may become possible to define one species similar to man, e.g. by pharmacokinetic behavior. If this were the best species available, we should consider performing routine chronic toxicity studies in this one species only, be it rodent or non-rodent. This in turn

Table 2. Information from chronic toxicity studies

Reason:	information on repeated dosing
	range finding for carcinogenicity
	range finding for reproduction
	range finding for mutagenicity
	control of pharmacological actions
	organ toxicity, behavior, hyperplasia, tumors
Describe:	morbidity > mortality
	dose response curve

Table 3. Aim of chronic toxicity studies

How: clinically, observation, weight, clinical chemistry, hematology, urinalysis, pathology, histology, target organs, behavior

Species: (1) 2 (1 rodent, 1 non-rodent)

Number: $\leqq 20\,(+5)$ rodents
$\qquad \leqq 4\,(+?)$ non-rodents

Route: (proposed)

Doses: (3) plus control

implies supportive (preliminary) studies in other species. Preliminary studies, independent of their purpose, should be performed with smaller numbers of animals.

Another problem is our approach to the number of animals used in routine studies. Why must 4 dogs be counterbalanced by 20 rodents per dose group and sex? On one hand, the number of animals is always too small to yield statistically "significant" and reliable results, on the other hand, models for semiquantitative evaluation of results obtained from small group of animals have been presented.

The number of species to be investigated in routine studies, the selection of species, and the number of animals to be used involve a vast amount of explosives for alternatives to classical chronic toxicity testing in the future.

Alternatives to and replacement of classical chronic toxicity studies

The classification and description of intentions have shown the refinements achieved during the last few years and those still pending. However, strategies to replace at least parts of the conventional studies have not yet been discussed. Therefore we have to look for different approaches, different systematization of our strategies dealing with chronic toxicity studies.

One such means is the description of the reasons for investigating toxicological risks in chronic studies. From charged or virtually haphazardous approaches to toxicology we have come to different and differential attempts.

It may become necessary to prove or disprove a suspicion, determine toxic concentrations at the target and to elucidate the mechanisms of toxic action. Such will be required to pursue development and/or clinical use of a drug which has given rise to suspicion because of routine investigations. It is understandable that the types of study to be performed now must differ – sometimes drastically – from routine protocols. It seems impossible to use one model experiment for all these purposes (Table 4).

Another scheme which might be useful in the search for alternatives to conventional routine chronic toxicity studies is the concept of *evidence* to be obtained (Table 5). This scheme contains a hierarchical order from estimation of a toxic potential (hazard) to risk estimation. While toxic potentials can be detected in whole animals or even lower organisms and subsystems, the results *per se* do not indicate their meaningfulness. Pharmacokinetic parameters can only be determined in whole animals (or using computers). Drug metabolism, however, can also be investigated *in vitro*. At least in mutagenicity studies we accept that the *in vivo* situation can be mimicked *in vitro* to yield meaningful results. Whether or not *in vitro* systems can be used routinely for the investigation of metabolic parameters in chronic toxicity studies requires further research. Information on the dose-response relationship can also be obtained by use of non-whole animal systems in order to better understand what was observed *in vivo*, whereas risk estimation has to consider all data collected.

It therefore becomes understandable that our dogma, that only chronic toxicity studies can give us the answer to chronic toxicity, is no longer valid. In contrast, we are in desperate need of additional information.

Modified intact whole animals are routinely used in pharmacology. Their use in toxicology, however, is rare. High blood pressure rats may be considered for the investigation of toxicity of antihypertensive agents, and diabetic animals for testing antidia-

Table 4. Reasons for investigating toxicological risks

- Routine investigation
- Proof or disproof of suspicion
- Determination of »toxic concentrations«
- Elucidation of mechanism of action

Table 5. Evidence to be obtained from chronic toxicity studies

- Toxic potential
- Pharmacokinetic parameters
- Dose response relationship
- Risk estimation

Table 6. Systems available for assessment of chronic toxicity

- Intact organism
- Modified intact organism
- Isolated organs
- Organ culture
- Tissue culture
- Cell culture
- Subcellular preparations

Table 7. Alternatives/Replacements/Additions to chronic toxicity testing in animals

- Number and selection of species
- Number of animals
- Number of experiments
- Number of additional investigations
- Mutual recognition

betic drugs. Besides such whole animal systems, subsystems are available (Table 6), which have proven useful for the investigation of the mode of toxic action and the solution of special problems of metabolism. Possible target organs can be used in cases of suspicion. The organs can be obtained from some extra animals added to routine studies, and special tests and experiments can be performed. A few additional tests are: physiological ones, EEC, and special morphological methods (morphometry, special staining techniques, electron microscopy, histochemistry, local reactions). Local reactions might even be studied in the same animals by administering the drug intravenously or intraarterially at the end of the study.

Conclusion

In summary, it can be stated that there is no real alternative to chronic toxicity testing. The problem of alternatives to chronic toxicity testing can and has been tackled by shaping the standard methods available today. This applies to the duration of studies, number and selection of species, number of animals as well as the total number of experiments required (Table 7). In addition to this conventional approach, other approaches have to be sought, but most of these will not be real alternatives in the truest sense of the word. A basic approach is the mutual recognition by the governmental institutions in the countries. Our European Notes for Guidance are open enough to accomodate future changes.

Reference

1. Repeated Dose Toxicity – Annex I (1983) Note for Guidance concerning the application of chapter I (B) (2) of part 2 of the Annex to Directive 75/318/EEC, with a view to the granting of a marketing authorization for a new drug. Official Journal of the European Communities, L 332, Vol 26, Nov 28 pp 12–19

Authors' address:
Dr. med. R. Baß
Institute for Drugs of the
Federal Health Office
Seestraße 10
D-1000 Berlin 65
F.R.G.

What good are clinical trials?

P. J. Fell

In fifteen years of conducting clinical trials, monitoring or reviewing them for medical journals there has been little change in the general pattern, some are good, some are poor, a few are excellent and thankfully very few are unethical or dangerous. The advances in medicine seem to have complicated the picture of clinical trials rather than simplified it and, as Peter Armitage says, each new trial has not put out the fires of controversy but has fanned them. I think one of the reasons for this is that more complex and difficult areas of therapy are being investigated and a more objective and scientific approach is being attempted, sometimes where this is most difficult. Whether a trial is excellent, of value or not, it has to be remembered each one involves patient care, the time of physicians and staff. Many require large amounts of money and other resources and therefore to make a judgement of how good they are will always be a question of balance, not only between benefit and risk but also between value in its widest sense and the resources expended.

Dilemmas

The scientific approach until replaced by better knowledge or new tools must be accepted as the only possibility for the majority of new investigations within medicine. Over-riding all are the ethical considerations which out-weigh all scientific restraints or instruments, and no matter how the work might benefit mankind generally or benefit future generations, the individual patient's rights are absolute. Therefore studies without a truly "informed consent" and an acceptable ethical review are not of any value, and it is essential that all clinical trials, no matter where they are conducted, in whichever country, should meet the minimum standard of ethical practice and fulfill the requirements of the Helsinki agreement.

Scientific method and physical science are absolute and measurements are accurate; however in medical science we must often approximate, and the degree of accuracy depends on the number of patients included. Thus the movement to greater accuracy demands a greater number of patients and this too may interfere or collide with the rights of an individual patient.

If ethics and medical care deem that a particular statistical or scientific approach is not possible then of course this may invalidate the clinical trial. Often tools can be found to ensure that a degree of scientific control is introduced without necessarily formally including statistics and many pilot studies indicating the value of a new drug can succeed by using careful observer techniques. Nevertheless there must occasionally be a trade-off, but never at the cost of sound ethical practice.

So the scientific and statistical aspects must be correct for a clinical trial to be of general value; consider first four aspects of the scientific method that Vere considers to be advantageous.

1. It gives the greatest ability to compare knowledge gained in different places at different times. It is "updatable".
2. It makes the detection and removal of bias including personal bias easier than any other method.
3. Its results are continuously corrigible because it works in corroboration and falsification of theories (Popper 1980).
4. It nevertheless allows (and should indeed encourage) that serendipity or inspiration without which new knowledge is meagre indeed, but does so without also allowing extravagance because it controls the input of such ideas into a system of knowledge by the mechanisms just mentioned.

Accepting these criteria and the ethical constraints we may now make judgements on the overall value of any clinical trial. On the other hand diseases are often not clearly diagnoseable, some have unusual presentations and some are insufficient in number to conduct a clinical trial. Often, as knowledge increases, more cases are recognised and therefore recording, particularly in surgery and new types of medical treatment of single cases, can be of value and used in future by other physicians and surgeons. We must not dismiss expert personal opinion, empiricism or restricted observation as valueless. It must however always be viewed with care and balanced against the present knowledge.

Nevertheless there are investigators who consider that randomisation and control should begin immediately one has a hypothesis regarding treatment. In 1983 Spodick suggested there should be no pilot studies and that any protocol concerning an investigative technique or research project should start with controlled randomised clinical studies. He felt this was important because otherwise it might influence the outcome of following studies and prompt a decision to proceed along certain lines at the expense of others. This to a certain extent is also supported in a paper on multiplicity by Tukey, who felt that the use of investigative tools prior to strictly controlled clinical trials with ethical constraints may predetermine the outcome and direct the analysis and design along certain set paths which might not necessarily be correct or beneficial.

Debates and designs

The day to day variations in individual patients as well as those between patients with the same condition are in most situations minimised by controlled trial designs. By increasing the number of patients studied, the time span investigated or using a crossover technique within patients many of the variables can be reduced and compensated for. Nevertheless in many diseases the actual presentation of the condition in the patient cannot be compensated for by statistical tools. Studies such as the Framingham Study produce not only a wealth of positive data but also raise questions about care and treatment of coronary heart disease and hypertension which would not have otherwise been discovered.

a) Clinical trials on pain

One of the areas which is extremely difficult to study and where the debate about design is constantly under review is the investigation of pain, whether it is in joints, cardiac, abdominal or whatever. The problem is that many studies have recorded a high placebo response. Anyone who has conducted a pain study will know that many factors other than the pain itself are influential – patients' well-being, depression, family and social environment, and sleep greatly influence the intensity of the pain. If one then adds the variability of the disease itself, e.g. in arthritic conditions which fluctuate, it is not surprising that there is great difficulty in showing clear differences between placebo and active substances and that it is impossible to show differences between two active treatments.

b) Clinical trials in hypertension

A second design and doubt which serves as an example is the study of hypertension and its outcome. Again, there is no doubt from the Framingham Study that high blood pressure influences the frequency of stroke and possibly myocardial infarct, and certainly other factors such as smoking have a clear effect. Consequently, the control of blood pressure is an important parameter and an essential part of patient care. Most studies that one is asked to review consist of comparisons with an active substance or in certain instances of mild hypertension with placebo conducted for several weeks and this shows a drug activity. It often does not show the drug in its correct light with respect to tolerability, control of blood pressure and outcome.

A few years ago we conducted a naturalistic study into the treatment of hypertension in an attempt to see how one or two particular drugs were used within our practice. The group studied was between twenty and sixty years of age and this amounted to 3,489 patients, of whom we managed to screen 3,222. After a careful assessment, 192 of these patients were found suitable for treatment of hypertension but subsequently only 138 were entered into the study. I do not want to dwell on the study too much, just to say at the outset that all blood pressures were collected under strict epidemiological conditions and the patients were seen on a regular basis by the same research nurses and doctors.

Two schedules were used (Table 1), one starting with a beta blocker, the other with a diuretic and increasing in potency first, then with combinations and finally a powerful hypotensive regime.

c) Blind observer techniques

The blind observer method used was that the doctor screened the patients and determined whether they were well controlled, with or without side effects, and could continue on a particular regime, or whether that level of treatment was unsuitable, in which case it should either be decreased or increased by the nurse changing the treatment by moving the schedule either up or down.

Of the 138 patients admitted to the study 84 completed treatment (Table 2). Over the two years 54 dropped out of the study for the reasons shown in Table 3, from Table 1

Table 1. Stabilizing treatment level of patients completing the study (Two blocks showing the majority of patients receiving blocker, diuretic or combination of the two – groups A, B, C, E, F)

Metoprolol starters				Chlorthalidone starters		
Male	Female	Totals		Male	Female	Totals
A = 10	A = 8	18		E = 7	E = 10	17
B = 4	B = 4	8		F = 6	F = 5	11
C = 7	C = 9	16		G = 2	G = 1	3
D1 = –	D1 = 2	2		H1 = –	H1 = 2	2
D2 = –	D2 = 1	1		H2 = –	H2 = 1	1
D3 = –	D3 = –	–		H3 = 2	H3 = 1	3
D4 = –	D4 = 1	1		H4 = –	H4 = 1	1
		46				38 = 84

Table 2. Patients completing the study

Male				Female				Total
50+	40+	30+	20+ Years	50+	40+	30+	20+ Years	
15	17	4	2	33	9	4	–	84

Table 3. Patients dropping out from the study

	Male				Female				Total
	50+	40+	30+	20+	50+	40+	30+	20+	
Schedule 1									
Uncooperative	1	1	–	–	4	1	–	–	
Hosp. tr.-g/away*	–	1	–	–	–	–	–	–	
Non responder		–	–	–	–	–	–	–	
Died	2	–	–	–	–	–	–	–	
Raynauds	1	1	–	–	2	1	1	–	
Side effects	–	1	–	–	4	1	–	–	
Normotensive	–	–	–	–	–	–	–	–	
Schedule 2									
Uncooperative	2	–	1	–	1	2	–	–	
Hosp. tr.-g/away*	–	–	–	–	1	2	–	–	
Non responder	–	–	–	–	1	–	–	–	
Died	–	–	–	–	–	–	–	–	
Raynauds	1	–	–	–	4	1	–	–	
Side effects	2	–	–	1	8	1	–	–	
Impotency	1	1	–	–	–	–	–	–	
Normotensive	1	–	–	–	–	–	–	–	
	12	5	1	1	25	9	1	–	54

* Hosp. tr.-g/away = Hospital transfer/gone away

one can see that the majority of patients moved only as far through the schedule as to require a beta blocker and a diuretic, that is at level C or level F. This would lead one to believe therefore, that such a combination would be suitable in the long term to control the majority of hypertensives within our practice.

Since that time this group of patients has been followed and of the 84 patients only 30 still remain on those particular combinations, having changed to other beta blockers or diuretics because of minor side effects or complaints by the patient.

The next example I should like to present is again from our work on hypertension. This particular study is in patients aged over 60 years who suffer from systolic hypertension with systolic blood pressure greater than 160 mm Hg and diastolic blood pressure less than 120 mm Hg, who have no other cardiovascular signs of symptoms and who otherwise would be deemed fit and well. We screened 1,480 patients in this age catagory and from these located 240 patients who would qualify. The study was such that they were either receiving placebo or beta blocker or diuretic plus beta blocker. Again all measurements were to a strict epidemiological protocol and these patients have now been followed for a total period of 9 years. We are currently producing our five-year results and there is one particular aspect I should like to present. Quite a number of patients over the five-year period demonstrated a fluctuation in blood pressure to such an extent that they fell well outside our criteria for admission and would be considered normotensive.

Many patients as would be expected receiving placebo demonstrated high systolic blood pressure. If you consider this particular patient (Fig. 1) who was one of many it will be noted that for a long period the patient was normotensive despite receiving placebo only. We log all consultations and complaints by the patient, and therefore can be quite assured that at these times there was no inter-current infection or other problem noted.

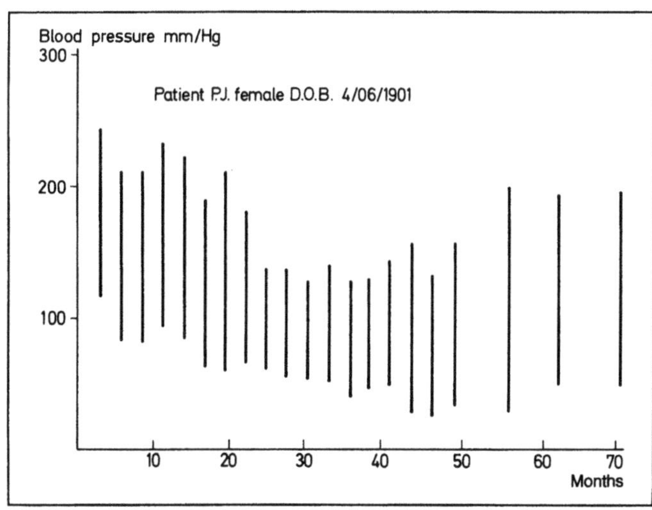

Fig. 1. Example of a patient receiving placebo during 70 week period: blood pressure results.

d) Extrapolation of clinical trials

Therefore it does appear that, contrary to our belief, patients over the age of 60 are still capable of having labile blood pressure and despite a screening period of six weeks, when the blood pressure remained above the 160 mmHg mark, they can for long periods of time be normotensive. Consequently, if this variable can alter slowly with time then it has a bearing on the type of treatment given. Any study which was conducted during a period of change would lead one to believe a drug to be effective in hypertension, but this is not the case. Therefore one should view clinical trials, particularly where such slow changes occur, with caution and not necessarily extrapolate results to long-term treatment from short-term studies.

e) Influential factors in clinical trials

The last area I should like to consider is where there are debates over design in clinical trials, as a result of other influences on outcome. Figure 2 shows that there are three important factors, the patient, disease and the drug; the combination of these determines the outcome of the condition and therefore these will be the three determinants which decide the success or failure of the clinical trial. There are many factors that influence all three, but also some which affect individual facets more than others.

i) General factors

Consider first the general factors (Fig. 2). The patients will influence the effect of the disease by their attitude towards it, and this includes factors such as acceptance, depression, will to overcome, discomfort etc. Equally the patient will have an effect on the drug by the degree of compliance and acceptance of the preparation, which is complicated by the physician who actually provides it. The disease and the morbidity it produces have a direct effect on the patient, and also produce a number of indirect ef-

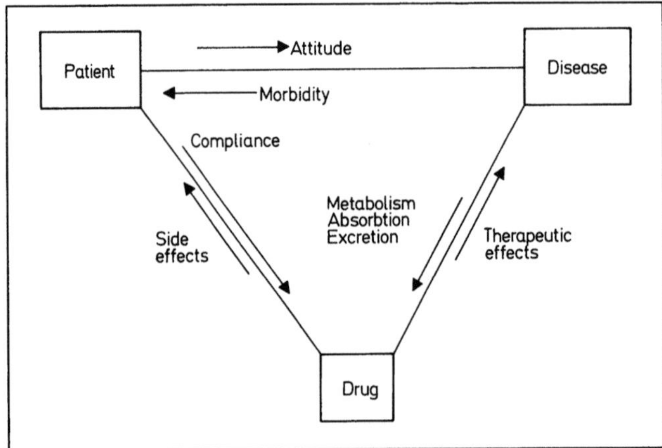

Fig. 2

32

fects on appetite, well-being etc. and may directly affect the drug by altering metabolism, absorption or excretion.

The drug in turn has an effect both on the patient with respect to side effects and the therapy, affecting, one hopes, the disease process.

If one now looks at each of these factors individually there are a number of things that affect the patient.

ii) The patient

Influencing factors are: the sleep pattern (if it becomes disturbed or a problem it may influence therapy), the mood of the patient, the family support that the patient is given, the degree of social activity or deprivation that the patient suffers as a consequence of the disease, and the effect of the drug as far as side effects are concerned on appetite etc. (Fig. 3).

An interesting example of the way that attitude can quite markedly affect outcome of a disease and its treatment is illustrated by some work conducted on breast cancer by Stephen Greer in 1979. From Table 4 you see that patients diagnosed as having breast cancer showed four types of response on psychological testing:

1. A denial, a refusal to accept the diagnosis
2. A fighting spirit.
3. A stoic acceptance.
4. A helplessness.

On the right hand side of the table you will note the five-year survival time 75% of points one and two whereas only 35% of points three and four survived 5 years. Therefore it is important to bear such conditions in mind and the powerful effect attitude may have on the outcome of a clinical study. "The amount of treatment received by 380 patients with back ache was found to have been influenced more by their distress and illness behaviour than by the actual physical disease. Patients showing a large amount of inappropriate illness behaviour had received significantly more treatment (p. .001)" (Waddell 1984).

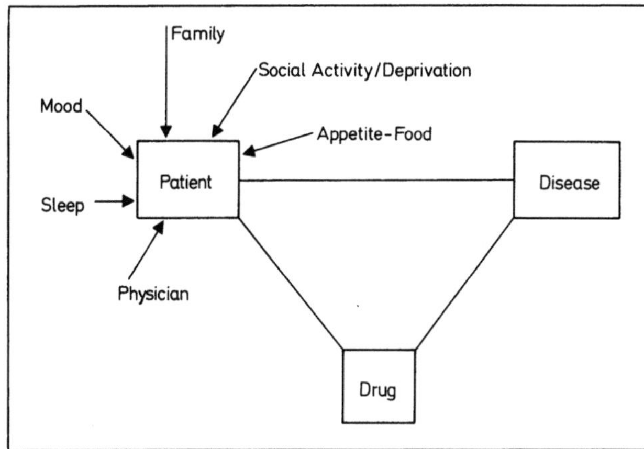

Fig. 3

Table 4. Psychological response to breast cancer – effect on outcome

Response	5 Yr. Survival
1. Denial (refusal to accept diagnosis)	75%
2. Fighting spirit (I can beat it)	
3. Stoic acceptance (I shall go on as normal)	35%
4. Helplessness (I am finished)	

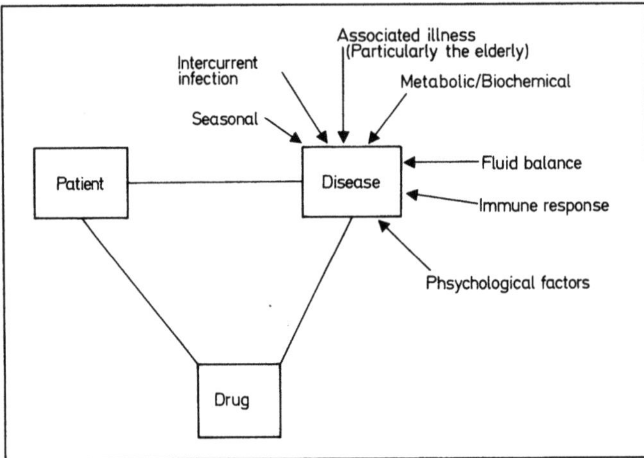

Fig. 4

There are therefore many factors other than the particular disease that must be taken into consideration.

iii) The disease (Fig. 4)

The disease on the other hand may be influenced by a number of outside factors not directly associated with the particular condition under treatment. This is particularly the case in elderly patients who may have a list of eight or nine pathologies, one of which is being considered in relation to a drug.

An associated illness, intercurrent infection, metabolic and biochemical changes, fluid balance, immune response, any psychological factors can actually affect the disease process. There also seem to be a number of seasonal factors which cannot be clearly defined but certainly cause an alteration of the disease process. This is obviously clear-cut in such allergic conditions as hay fever or where a particular cause of the disease is seasonal, but there are also many other factors such as weather, length of day etc. which have perhaps to be studied in detail.

Finally we come to effects which have been known to cause alteration in the way the drug is accommodated.

34

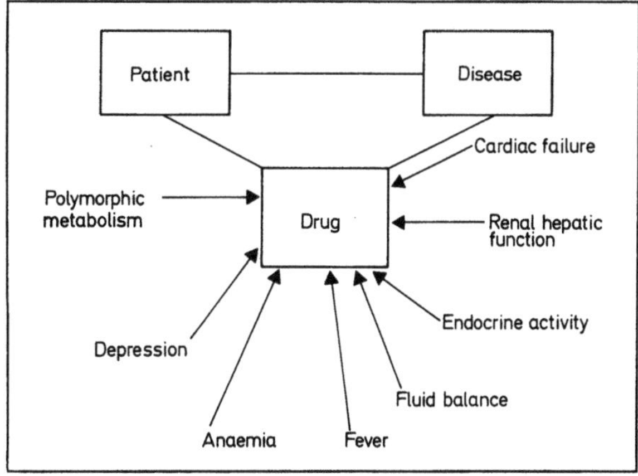

Fig. 5

iv) The drug (Fig. 5)

Degree of cardiac failure can effect many treatments, renal and hepatic function, endocrine activity and fluid balance, the effect of a fever can alter absorption and distribution of a drug as can anaemia. The problems of depression can actually suppress the effects of certain anti-inflammatory and pain killing drugs. More recently, we have become aware of the very exciting and important effect of polymorphic metabolism and the genetic make-up of the patient which directly affect the way drugs may be metabolised.

This particular aspect of acceptability and adverse drug reaction in patients is yet to be proven, and only small studies have been conducted showing a direct influence of polymorphic metabolism on particular drugs.

Therefore, knowing that there are many outside factors which can influence the outcome of a clinical trial it is not always possible to ensure that the design will embrace all factors. However, by using randomisation one can hopefully ensure that a reasonable distribution of variables occurs between drug and comparative substance and stratification can be used where clear-cut problems can be looked on as subgroups of an overall study. The multiplicity within a study where different timing and responses variables are considered within one particular clinical trial should be taken into account. Many of these factors by the very use of numbers can be minimised, but equally in studies that are combined and multiplied they can appear to be a problem. Interestingly a paper by Lewis in 1982 surveyed 29 trials that had been conducted using a beta blocker and its effect on secondary prevention of myocardial infarction. These studies were quite differently designed with different drugs, admission criteria spread over several centers, investigators, etc. Nevertheless it was possible using a pooling technique to show some quite remarkable results. This is often not even the case within one set of clinical trails for one particular drug. It cannot therefore be generally applied, but the more it could be the better, as it decreases the amount of work and number of patients to be studied.

Conclusion

Karl Popper (1959) noted "Once put forward none of our anticipations are dogmatically upheld. Our method of research is not to defend them to prove how right they are, on the contrary we try to overthrow them."
Medical education is a structured learning of an art and science applied by an individual or team who themselves have an influence on the disease process. Also, the patient's acceptance and belief many influence the outcome. So to overthrow these is often impossible for some physicians and difficult for most.
The problem is further compounded; scientific discipline which is contrary to medicine being applied in clinical practice.
Again referring back to one of our studies of patients over 60 with systolic hypertension, a piece of dogma that I believe we accepted was that this particular patient age-group changed very little. Therefore, treatment once established and well tolerated will be unlikely to change or be stopped.
In Table 5 you can see the number of patients who were washed out of their treatment, and you will note quite a considerable proportion, 27, were able to stop therapy, and indeed for several years of follow-up remained off treatment.
Thus it is very important to test our theories and hypotheses regularly to ensure that we are conforming to Popper's statement.
On balance the scientific approach to therapeutics in various forms has been successful and produced major advances. These advances may in comparison be overshadowed by the events that occurred earlier this century when combating poor hygiene and social deprivation caused a major decline in many diseases such as tuberculosis and rheumatic fever. Nevertheless, the new antibiotics, steroids and oral contraceptives, the control of cardiovascular disease and hypertension without crippling side effects, the safer control of depression and psychotic illness have all been the result of good sound clinical trial work and have stood the test of time.
The results of well applied regulations were initially of great value and sucessful in preventing serious side effects of new drugs. However, they have still allowed drugs to reach the market which do have detrimental effects, and the adoption of a very restrictive attitude has if anything induced an increase in unnecessary trials and sometimes prevented the early use of new and useful compounds.
The industry cannot escape criticism either in its urgency to enter therapeutic areas which appear lucrative and occasionally by taking short cuts has produced not only poor clinical trial work but also managed to market compounds which have later been proved to be either unsatisfactory or unsafe.

Table 5. Washout

Uncooperative	1
Unsuitable after complete or washout	36
Normotensive	27
Proceeded to trial	22
Total	85

Not withstanding these comments we still need new therapy for many areas of medicine. Many of the existing drugs for important pathological states are still inadequate or carry with them serious side effects. Consequently, new trial work in more difficult areas will be necessary. Furthermore, long-term studies to gain more insight into the natural history of disease and its relationship to drugs require complex statistical analysis and careful monitoring. Perhaps therefore in many areas new approaches should be encouraged. A more cautious approach, initially to ensure that safety aspects of the drug are proven, followed by a wider exploratory role in the clinical phases, should be encouraged. This may lead to drugs being used in fewer patients in clinical trials and reaching the market earlier. If this were followed by a more careful surveillance during phase three and early marketing it might be possible to enlarge the therapeutic arsenal without necessarily causing the patients to be at risk. Having looked at a number of aspects of clinical trials I think one can say that the controlled clinical trial is at present the only tool we have for new drug investigation which can stand scientific scrutiny. Therefore it is of use, and if correctly and sensibly applied with insight and consideration to the patient and the ethical aspects of medicine it is a valuable tool.

Lastly I would like to leave you with a rather cynical look (Fig. 6) at what good are clinical trials.

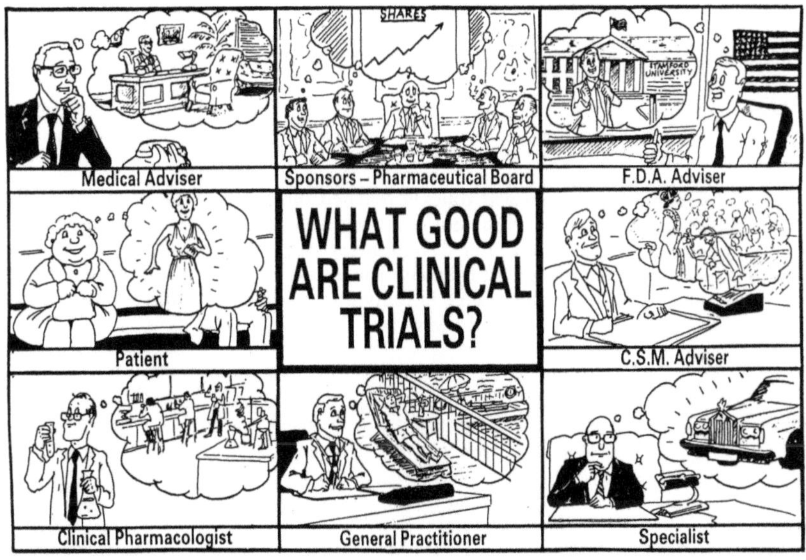

Fig. 6

References

1. Armitage P (1984–85) Controversy and Achievements in Clinical Trials. Controlled Clinical Trials p 67–72
2. Greer S (1979) Psychological Response to Breast Cancer, effect on outcome. Lancet 2:785–787
3. Fell PJ et al (1982) The Naturalistic Study of Hypertension – 2 year results. Eur J Clin Pharmacol

4. Kannel WB, Sorlie P et al (1975) Hypertension in Framingham. In: Payl O (ed) Epidemiology and Control of Hypertension. Symposia Specialists, Miami, p 553–592
5. Lewis JA (1982) Beta Blockade After Myocardial Infarct. Br J Clin Pharmacol 14:15–21
6. Popper K (1959) The Logic of the Scientific Discovery. Hutchinson, London
7. Popper K (1980) The Logic of Scientific Discovery (rev 10th impression) Hutchinson, London, pp 16, 30–32, 41, 149–150, 167–169
8. Spodick DH (1983) Randomise the First Patient: Scientific, Ethical and Behavioral Bases. Am J Cardiol 51:p 916–917
9. Tuckey JW (1977) Multiplicity. Science p 198
10. Vere D (1982) Scientific Philosophy Applied to Clinical Medicine. Expentia (suppl) vol 41:28–34
11. Waddell G (1984) Symptoms and signs: physical disease or illness behaviour? Br Med J 289:739–742

Authors' address:
Dr. Peter J. Fell
Deddington Health Center
Earls Lane,
Deddington.
Oxfordshire OX5 4TQ, Great Britain

Discussion

FELL:
In the discussion of this paper agreement was quickly reached on the importance of conducting careful dose-range studies early in the development of a drug. It was further stressed that one still has to keep a careful eye on dosage during later development stages and even after the drug has reached the market. Finally, it was pointed out that with some drugs (e.g. many antihypertensives) the correct medical practice is to titrate the dosage in individual patients and that this therapeutic fact of life should and can be reflected in clinical trials.

Clinical guidelines – a help or a hindrance?

M. N. G. Dukes

However far science and medicine progress, they never quite seem to escape from the shadow of the Tower of Babel. Linguistic confusion continues to succeed, now and again, in thwarting their deliberations and obscuring their aims. The issue of Guidelines for the Clinical Investigation of Drugs is a case in point. They are hailed by some and condemned by others and nine tenths of the problem is that the one party really has little idea what the other party is talking about.

If I were asked to say what the term Guideline conveys to me, as someone whose native language was once English, then I would probably answer that a guideline is something more than a casual suggestion and much less than a binding command. At its best, I think one could consider a guideline to be a well thought out piece of advice on the best way to undertake a job, taking into account current knowledge. The user will be well advised to read it but there is no obligation on him to follow it; it simply indicates the state of the art at the moment that it is drawn up, as perceived by a number of well-informed and hopefully wise people.

So far, so good. The trouble is, of course, that in Europe we speak several dozen languages, and we have grown up with as many different legal traditions. In some languages, guidelines are quite simply guidelines in the English sense. In Scandinavia we speak of "rettningslinjer", which is exactly the same word; similarly we find "Richtlinie" in German and "richtlijn" in Dutch. Beyond that we are rather lost. The European Community very soon found that in French there was no concept in between the mere "recommendation" and the stern "directive". Similarly at WHO in Copenhagen, with Russian as the most widely spoken language in our member states we had to choose between "rekomendatsii" and "ukazii"; there was no golden mean.

This goes at least part of the way to explaining why the debate about Guidelines for the Clinical Investigation of various groups of drugs has been so confused. The one sees in a guideline for such a purpose a mere opinion, which he suspects has cost a lot of the taxpayer's money to get down on paper. The other sees in a guideline some sort of dreadful edict which will tie him down for evermore, forbidding him to think for himself and paralyzing progress.

Guidelines for the Clinical Investigation of Drugs began to appear, in one form or another, as Clinical Pharmacology and the science of Clinical Investigation grew up in the 1950s and 1960s. One of the best examples was the still widely used blue booklet issued by the World Health Organization in 1968, known as "Principles for the Clinical Evaluation of Drugs". By present standards it is vague and full of truisms, but by the standards of 1968 it was a pioneering piece of work because it quite simply represented the first worldwide consensus document on the way that drugs should be examined in man. It helped to guide in the way that a guideline should, and it was undoubtedly one of the basic elements in putting clinical investigation of drugs into some semblance of order during the decade which followed.

Even at that time it was quite clear, however, that there was a need to go further. There were some very considerable differences between the methods used in examining an antidepressant drug and those applicable to a study of a topical corticosteroid cream. At the very least there were in each specific field of study a number of special pitfalls to be avoided which had been identified as a result of unfortunate experience and which needed putting down on paper, so that others would not continue to fall into the same errors. Obviously, however, many of these things were finding their way into the journals and books, both in original publications and reviews, and you can perfectly well put the question, now as then, whether there was any need for official bodies or international organizations to concern themselves with such details.

I will come back to the question as to whether such bodies should become involved in such matters. The point I must make at the moment is that for one reason or another they did, and it is interesting to look back and see why they did it.

The Drug Regulatory Agencies were first on the scene with guidelines for individual product groups. Very often, the famous series of investigational guidelines issued by the American FDA in the 1970s are cited as if they were the first and the best, but this perhaps refects nothing more than the fact that the FDA was at that time an agency with a great deal of international prestige. But it was not the first to publish a guideline by any means. The first, to my knowledge, was the Netherlands, which issued guidelines of the same type from 1964 onwards – just twenty years ago. The second was the Soviet Union, whose drug regulatory agency published guidelines from 1968 onwards. That these three pioneering agencies worked largely in isolation from one another was again a consequence of the language problem and the lack of contact between regulatory agencies which pertained twenty years ago until WHO in the early 1970s broke the deadlock with its annual regulatory conferences. In retrospect the surprising thing is that these guidelines had so many elements in common.

Just why these agencies came to issue guidelines for the clinical investigation of various groups of drugs is a matter on which I should dwell for a moment. Quite simply, all three were faced with a large number of companies applying for drug licences, some of which had very odd ideas as to how clinical research should be conducted. I do not think that anyone who has had a number of years of experience in drug regulation will be likely to dispute that statement. The quality of the work submitted as part of regulatory files is extraordinarily variable, and when it is not of a scientifically acceptable standard it is a frustrating exercise for all parties. My own personal experience was with the Committee for Evaluation of Medicines in the Netherlands, where detailed clinical guidelines had been in use for eight years at the time I joined the Committee, and there was no doubt that both the Committee and the drug industry found them useful as an outline of what the Committee would be likely to regard as adequate clinical work in any particular field. On some occasions the drug industry itself took the initiative to ask that a standard be agreed upon. One such case was with respect to non-steroidal anti-inflammatory agents, when several manufacturers, exasperated at being unable to meet the Committee's wishes regarding long-term studies, asked us to define them in clear terms. One of the results was a rather arbitrary minimum standard; at the time of application for a new drug licence, such a product must have been thoroughly tested for at least a year in at least a hundred patients. The standard was not rigidly enforced

40

but it was exactly what some medical directors had asked for – a target at which they could aim.

The above example brings me to the question of the legal status of a guideline issued by a regulatory committee. In Holland, quite clearly, our guidelines had no legal status at all; they were guidelines in the best sense of the word, helpful definitions of the state of the art which did not bind either party. That was not the case everywhere. In the Soviet Union, the guidelines for the evaluation of specific groups of drugs were very much a set of instructions which the applicant was obliged to follow in the course of his clinical investigation if he wished to have any hope of obtaining a drug licence. In the United States the position was again different; the guidelines issued by the F.D.A. had yet another status; they did and still do bind the agency, in the sense that it is obliged to accept a drug which meets the standards set out in the guideline, but they do not bind the manufacturer; if he wishes to try his luck with another mode of clinical investigation which he considers equally valid or superior he is free to do so.

Around the beginning of the 1970s then, and without having had any substantial contact with one another, these three agencies – in the Netherlands, the USA and the USSR – had all instituted regulatory guidelines for the clinical investigation of drugs belonging to the main therapeutic groups, though only the American guidelines ever became very widely known outside their own frontiers. A very few other agencies had issued guidelines for one or two isolated groups of products. At that point, however, several international developments started.

The first of these, although most people will I suspect have forgotten the fact, was the adaptation of some of Holland's guidelines for use by the new and short-lived Joint Benelux Service for Drug Registration, which existed only from 1973 to 1978 in its original form. It may have had no lasting significance, but it did develop the guideline tradition in Belgium and Luxemburg, and when five years later Leon Robert of Luxemburg became Chairman of the EEC's Committee for Proprietary Medicinal Products it was he who proposed that the EEC should follow the same course. And indeed a Working Group did develop so-called "Notes for Guidance of Applicants", several of which related to specific clinical areas; two of these – covering fixed combination products and nonsteroidal anti-inflammatory agents – were issued last year; several others went into the formal EEC procedure for approval and publication which is a relatively slow matter. The EEC Working Party, like the Dutch Committee before it, held hearings with the pharmaceutical industry before finalizing any text and took industry's views very seriously into account.

However, almost at the same time there was another development. In 1978 an Advisory Committee of the World Health Organization's Regional Office for Europe in Copenhagen proposed that, in view of the success of WHO's basic guideline for investigators of 1968, a number of supplementary documents should be drawn up by experts to give guidance in some specific investigational areas; hypotension was taken as the first of these, and a WHO Guideline was published in 1979; it was quite widely reproduced in the literature.

It is probably fair to say that at that point the wires became crossed. What happened was that the European Community's Committee on Proprietary Medicinal Products took the first of the WHO/EURO guidelines and accepted it for use as one of its own. At first sight one might conclude that this was very laudable, because it avoided the risk of discrepancies arising. In actual fact, I am not sure that it was a good thing. The WHO document, like those which followed it, was intended purely as a piece of well thought out advice written by investigators for investigators, and capable of being revised and updated very rapidly if the need arose. In Brussels it was introduced into an unavoidable bureaucratic machine where texts carry some sort of regulatory aura simply by virtue of the body which adopts them, and where changes and updating are not likely to be simple matters. Whether the EEC is likely to do the same with more recent WHO Guidelines is not clear; eleven have appeared to date, either in definitive or final draft form, so there is plenty of room for experiment.

I was asked to discuss the question as to whether clinical guidelines are a help or a hindrance, and I would now like to try and answer that question directly.

That they can often be a help is something one can judge quite simply by looking into the files in our own offices. We have received many hundreds of reactions, either from experts whom we consulted or from experts or bodies writing to us spontaneously. The overwhelming view is that there is a tremendous need for such documents. The reasons given tend to be very consistent. We receive for example many letters from professional associations welcoming consensus documents of this type, and in some cases offering to sponsor them. The European League Against Rheumatism is for example the sponsor of our Antirheumatic Guidelines, and an international society for cataract studies is sponsoring a guideline with us on drugs claimed to prevent or alleviate cataract. Individual investigators write to us that they welcome some clarity in this field, in which one can find so many conflicting opinions. As for their effects on the level of clinical investigation, I would like to quote the prestigious national medical research organization of one of our Western member states which wrote quite spontaneously to WHO a few weeks ago that it had identified a number of fields in which the standard of clinical studies was, to use its own words "not merely bad, but appalling". That particular organization had planned to develop its own clinical guidelines to do something about it, but now welcomed the chance of linking up with WHO to produce an international document. These views, and they are quite typical, leave no doubt at all that there is a real and widespread need for clinical investigational guidelines. Naturally there are some voices to the contrary; we received a letter a month ago from a very highly respected industrial source, arguing that our guidelines were of no conceivable use, a negative point of view, but one which stands almost alone in our files; the pharmaceutical industry is indeed among the sponsors of our WHO Guidelines and plays a very active role in producing them with us, and that is just as it should be.

Whether clinical guidelines can be a hindrance or not depends partly, I believe, on the body which produces them. Having experienced at first hand various of the developments which I have just talked about at the national, subregional, regional and global level, I might just as well admit to having acquired a very strong preference for guidelines to be developed by a non-regulatory health organization like WHO rather than by regulatory agencies. One of my main reasons for saying this is that, with science being constantly on the move, a guideline can and must be no more than the glimpse of a moment in time, a mile-post if you like on the road along which clinical research is developing. We have to avoid turning the mile-post into a barrier to progress, and that is the risk of defining our standards in legal and regulatory terms. WHO is well equipped to ensure that documents like this do represent a broad consensus between regulators, that they are produced and issued much more rapidly than is possible in a regulatory organization, and that they are updated whenever the need arises.

42

I am not of course now suddenly denying that there will be some need for regulatory documents as well, but these are more likely to be brief outlines of standards; a true clinical investigational guideline is likely to be discursive, explaining why some techniques are better than others but leaving the final approach to the investigator himself. The differences emerge very clearly if you contrast the EEC's Notes for Guidance on Non-Steroidal Anti-inflammatory agents – which in typewritten form run to three pages – with the WHO Guidelines on Antirheumatic Drugs which run to over forty. The documents are simply not comparable, but the difference between them is entirely defensible; a scientific guide to this complex field running to only three pages would be absurdly superficial, but, conversely, a regulatory document running to forty-odd pages would be a disaster for everyone.

In summary: there turns out to be a very considerable and proven demand for a series of global consensus documents, drawn up by experienced clinical investigators, on current approaches to the investigation of drugs in the main therapeutic areas, old and new. I submit that in the light of present experience one should look very carefully at the series of guidelines now appearing regularly from WHO's Copenhagen Office as candidates for that role. They have been produced at the suggestion of a wide range of sponsors variously including member states, professional associations, pharmaceutical companies and some of WHO's Global Programmes in Geneva or elsewhere. They are astonishingly low-cost products, particularly in view of their frequent sponsorship. They have been drawn up by groups of experts in each specific field, and submitted for comment to many hundreds of others, as well as to the pharmaceutical industry and the main regulatory bodies both within Europe and beyond. There has been close and cordial collaboration with two of three sub-regional organizations within the European region, namely the Comecon and the Nordic Council, and we all hope that the third of the sub-regional organizations, namely the European Community, will in due course respond to our many invitations to join in the project, rather than misconstrue it as competition to its own rather different and more limited activities.

Some people will always misunderstand and misuse whatever is put on paper as to the right way to conduct clinical studies, but there has fortunately been very little misunderstanding of this particular venture, at least among those who have examined this project and these documents at first hand. As a rule they have become enthusiastic and have joined in to help us. We extend an invitation to all of you to do the same.

Author's address:
Dr. M. N. G. Dukes
World Health Organization
8, Scherfigsvei
DK-2100 Copenhagen
Denmark

Discussion

DUKES:
Dr Dukes's remarks were followed by a lively discussion, comments from the floor being universally critical towards the production of clinical trial guidelines by WHO. First, it was suggested that WHO was the wrong organization to address this matter and should rather concentrate on the enormous health problems around the world. Second, the need for standardized guidance on how to conduct clinical trials was questioned and it was thought to be more important to harmonize regulatory requirements around the world. Third, specific criticisms of individual guidelines were voiced and the clinical expertise of the expert committee was questioned. Last, but by no means least, everyone at the discussion expressed concern that the WHO guidelines could be intellectually stultifying and would predictably not be interpreted by regulatory authorities as flexible guidelines but as statutory instruments. The speaker sought to allay these fears and suggested that specific criticisms of any guideline be put forward forcefully for consideration.

Clinical trials in the natural environment

Louis Lasagna

Introduction

In the last 40 years there has been a radical change in the ways of obtaining information about therapeutic agents that are considered valid by the scientific establishment and by national regulatory authorities. We have witnessed the ascendancy of the randomized, double-blind, controlled clinical trial (RCCT), to the point where many in positions of authority now believe that data obtained via this technique should constitute the only basis for registering a drug, or indeed for coming to any conclusions about its efficacy at any time in the drug's career. My thesis is that this viewpoint is untenable, needlessly rigid, unrealistic, and at times unethical.

Advantages and deficiencies of controlled trials

Let me begin, however, by paying tribute to the RCCT. I have been designing and executing such trials for over 30 years. Early in my academic career, I spent time writing and talking about the need for RCCTs, trying to convince others of their importance. My present position is by no means a rejection of the RCCT, but rather an appreciation both of what it can do, and what it cannot do. For some purposes, the RCCT is unexcelled. If one wants to convince the editors of journals, or regulatory authorities, or academics that a drug has the unquestioned ability to lower blood pressure, or help insomniacs to sleep, or relieve pain, or achieve almost any desired effect, be it subjective or objective, the experimental method, with its appropriate controls, is hard to beat. Having admitted that, I must go on to point out that for many other purposes, the RCCT is not indispensable and at times is not even useful.

Historical basis for controlled trials

Why has the RCCT achieved its current sanctified status? I believe that the explanation lies in three separate arenas. The first is a counter-reaction to the errors of the past, to the homage paid over the centuries by the sick and by the medical profession to false therapeutic idols – to moss from the skull of hanged criminals, to unicorn horn, to eunuch fat, to thousands of pseudo-remedies that are now thoroughly discredited.
The second factor is the growing appreciation of "the power of the placebo." While many still do not appreciate its double components – psychological anticipation and spontaneous change – the fact that therapeutic benefit can be erroneously attributed to entities without intrinsic pharmacodynamic activity cannot be denied. It makes no dif-

ference that in most trials – indeed almost without exception – one cannot tease out the psychological component from the spontaneous change component. For purposes of avoiding the error of misattribution of pharmacodynamic effect, the placebo is an admirable analogue of the chemist's "blank."

The third factor was the evolution of statistics away from the simple counting of events such as births, deaths, congenital anomalies, infectious diseases, etc. – so-called "vital statistics" – and towards techniques for estimating probability and for extrapolating from samples of the population of interest to the larger universe of potential subjects. This statistical revolution provided the foundation for the analyses and setting of confidence limits that we take for granted today as an inevitable part of the experimental method.

Discoveries through observation

While it is true that older observational (nonexperimental) techniques could lead one into error, it is also true that most valid medical knowledge has resulted from shrewd observation and analysis by a keen physician or scientist ready to profit from what he saw. As Pasteur said, "Chance favors only the prepared mind." Our pathology texts are testimony to observation, as are our surgical texts. Withering was able to appreciate with remarkable accuracy the wonders and the side effects of digitalis, and gave splendid directions for its use, without having ever heard of randomization and the double-blind. Nor were modern trial techniques necessary to recognize the therapeutic potential of chloral hydrate, the barbiturates, ether, nitrous oxide, chloroform, curare, aspirin, quinine, insulin, thyroid, epinephrine, local anesthetics, belladonna, antacids, sulfonamides, and penicillin, to give a partial list.

I do not suggest that worshippers of the RCCT deny the past, but they quite properly ask, "How is one to know whether one is dealing with a true remedy or a false one, when the course of most ills is so variable and unpredictable?" The answer to that, I submit, is that it is possible for observations to err as well as to come to correct conclusions, but the same can be said for a RCCT, which can be plagued by Type II error because it studied the wrong patients, or too few of them, or used the wrong dose or incompetent investigators.

In addition, I am persuaded that our ability to discriminate true therapeutic effect from false has been greatly enhanced by the availability in modern times of remedies of proven merit. When only trivially effective remedies are available to treat a disease or a symptom, the physician's judgment about a new remedy is more likely to be faulty than when he has had a chance to observe the impact of truly effective drugs.

Other failings of controlled trials

I have mentioned some of the ways by which a RCCT can come to grief. Let us examine some of its other failings. While it is relatively simple to assign available patients randomly to the treatments under scrutiny, it is quite literally *never* possible to study a random sample of the *universe* of patients in the ultimate target population. Hence we are always left, after a trial, with the nagging worry that our results are not necessarily capable of extrapolation to other patients. This problem existed even before modern society began to demand that informed consent be obtained from experimental subjects, but new ethical constraints have made further inroads on recruitment and possibly hampered even further our attempts to generalize.

But even within the population studied, the RCCT is usually less useful than we would like it to be in providing the practicing doctor with specific advice. The RCCT is usually employed to demonstrate what I like to call "the herd phenomenon," i.e., to show that in a given *group* of patients the drug was *on average* better than placebo. The focus is on demonstrating a statistically significant effect in the group, *not* the individual. (Sometimes the effect is biologically trivial, but that is a separate problem.)

The needs of individual patients

This situation is, of course, the antithesis of the practice of medicine, where the focus is on the *individual,* who does not care if a drug is safe and effective for others if it fails so to perform for him. It is fascinating how few formal attempts have been made to "fine tune" the use of a drug, although the literature contains a large number of retrospective analyses of trials that seemingly have identified patient factors that affected the nature or degree of response to a drug. While some of these post hoc correlations are almost certainly spurious, others are not, and our ability to identify these factors in advance should increase our ability to tailor the choice of drug, and its regimen, to the needs of individual patients. Our efforts to do so, however, are not helped by the unfortunate tendency of protocol designers to employ fairly rigid dosage schedules for logistic reasons.

Currently unmet needs

If we now ask what we often do *not* know about a drug when it is registered, it will become even more apparent why careful observations will be necessary after registration. For we will want to know the answers to questions such as the following:

What is the effect of kidney disease on drug response? Of liver disease? Of coadministered prescription or over-the-counter drugs?

What special risks are run by pregnant women and their unborn fetuses? By pediatric patients? By the elderly?

Will the drug be abused? What is the clinical picture in cases of gross overdosage, accidental or purposeful?

What will be the effect on the drug's performance of capricious compliance with prescribing directions? Of the involvement of physicians less expert than those who studied the drug prior to registration?

How can we identify the very rare but serious side effect? The long-delayed side effect?

Surely the answers to the above are not likely to derive from RCCTs. History also teaches us that the drug doses recommended at the time of initial marketing on the basis, largely, of RCCTs may need to be revised on the basis of post-registration experience of the "naturalistic" variety. (It is not only surgeons who learn to perform an operation better with experience, and to choose their patients for the operation with more skill; prescribers of drugs have a similar possibility of improving their performance.) Sometimes recommended drug dosages are revised upwards, sometimes downward, as a result of experience.

Ethical problems will also have to be faced. Placebo controls are increasingly difficult to defend as better drugs are developed. Patients in different countries may respond differently to the same drug, for reasons of genetics, nutrition, or what have you. But must this possibility be checked out with duplicative RCCTs, or can we use naturalistic experience by competent physicians using as a basis the data accumulated by their peers in other lands?

Recent proposals for reconsidering present attitudes

It is of interest that distinguished figures have recently been speaking out in favor of a more tolerant attitude toward clinical experiences. Thus Bailar et al. (1984) have said, "In spite of potential pitfalls, carefully selected and reported studies without internal controls can play a substantial part in the acquisition of scientific knowledge." The eminent statistician, Lincoln E. Moses, looking back on such uncontrolled series of cases as John Snow's 75 operations under ether anesthesia and Pierre Louis's 77 patients with pneumonia who were bled to no purpose, has said, "A series study is a record of experience; as such it has prima facie value. It may give very useful information. . . ." (Moses 1984).

John D. Archer (1984) has lately pointed out many important uses of drugs that have been discovered post-registration and often by observation rather than experiment. Indeed some of these new uses were for diseases actually considered *contraindications* prior to the ultimate triumph of truth over error! Archer's list includes propranolol for angina pectoris and hypertension, metronidazole for amebiasis, amantadine for Parkinsonism and the treatment of A_2 influenza, diazepam for status epilepticus, imipramine for childhood enuresis, cholestyramine resin for hyperlipidemia, and lidocaine for arrhythmias.

It is for all these reasons that I have labelled as both silly and anti-intellectual those who would ignore or decry naturalistic medical experience. Such people belittle the practice of medicine and deny to the physician the benefit of his own patient encounters. As I have said, "The intelligent physician will apply [historical] controls while being wary of their deficiencies (Lasagna 1982)."

It is bizarre that regulators and others are so willing to accept naturalistic experience when it comes to adverse effects, but not when it involves benefit. Why? Surely misattribution of toxicity can be as serious as misattribution of benefit.

In 1965, Sir Austin Bradford Hill, a leader in the early development of controlled trials, said in his Heberden Oration: "Given the right attitude of mind, there is more than one way in which we can study therapeutic efficacy. Any belief that the controlled trial is the only way would mean not that the pendulum had swung too far but that it had come right off its hook (Hill 1966)."

To that, one can only add: "Amen."

References

1. Bailar JC III, Louis TA, Lavori PW, Polansky M (1984) Studies without internal controls. New Engl J Med 311:156–162
2. Moses LE (1984) The series of consecutive cases as a device for assessing outcomes of intervention. New Engl J Med 311:705–710
3. Archer JD (1984) The FDA does not approve uses of drugs. JAMA 252:1054–1055
4. Lasagna L (1982) Historical controls – the practitioner's clinical trials. New Engl J Med 307:1339–1340
5. Hill AB (1966) Heberden Oration, 1965. Reflections on the controlled trial. Am Rheum Dis 25:107–113

Author's address:
Louis Lasagna, M.D.
Tufts University
Boston, Mass. 02111
U.S.A.

Discussion

LASAGNA:
One person present felt that the speaker had given the impression that herbal medicines were probably no better than placebos. He reminded the audience that many important modern drugs had originated from plant medicines. He urged that plant products used in folklore medicine be investigated with modern methods. The speaker fully agreed with this view. He suggested that an interesting approach might to be begin with plant remedies that had been used in widely separated geographical areas for the same therapeutic purpose.

Clinical trials and the general practitioner

Paolo E. Lucchelli

Introduction

The process of clinical development of a new drug has so far involved the general practitioner (GP) only to a very marginal extent. Obvious safety reasons and, at least in Italy, the law prevent the GP from taking a direct part in the first phases of clinical research; on the other hand, even after the introduction of a medicine onto the market, the general practitioner's involvement is considered to be that of prescription rather than evaluation.

Yet the participation of the general practitioner in a late phase of a drug evaluation programme can be justified both theoretically and practically despite the methodological and operational problems involved. Such problems are particularly evident in the so-called "extensive" clinical trials, i.e. studies involving many or even hundreds of doctors in various locations, whereas when the number of doctors involved is smaller, the problems are more similar to those of a traditional clinical study, the difference being essentially in the difficulties of direct and frequent monitoring.

Why should trials be performed in general practice?

The real testing bench for many drugs is general practice. Currently a large amount of information that could be used to better define a drug profile is wasted because a systematic approach to GPs' clinical observations is lacking.

In fact, by the end of Phase 3, a fairly accurate knowledge of a drug has been obtained, which in general statistical terms can be defined as the availability of a number of mean values and their confidence limits. However there is now a general consensus that the artificial environment of formal clinical trials does not necessarily show exactly how the drug will behave in all the eventualities occurring in everyday general practice.

Patients in their own surroundings may respond differently to a drug in terms both of efficacy and tolerability. Wheatley (1973) reported on this aspect in the first International Meeting of Pharmaceutical Physicians, and it is discussed by Lasagna in this book. Suffice it to mention the different severity levels of disease, the various degrees of importance that a side effect, for example drowsiness, can assume in the hospital and at work and the greater difficulty in following complex dosage schedules at home. Moreover, in the everyday world outside the hospital, "extrapharmacological" factors, such as packaging and tablet shape, colour and flavour all play a role in determining the general acceptability of the product. Last but not least, rarer adverse reactions emerge only after extensive use of the drug in everyday life.

What could be done in a general practice trial?

There is an area in Phases 2 and 3 in which the intervention of general practitioners could be the determining factor in the success or failure of a trial. There are studies in which the patients enrolled have to attend hospital out-patient departments for visits as required by the protocol, but in the intervals between these visits a patient is generally under the care of his family doctor: the latter can thus make an important contribution by checking that the patient complies with the instructions received; however it sometimes happens that, due to a lack of coordination between the research centre and the GP, instead of collaborating the practitioner develops an indifferent or even hostile attitude: in extreme cases he may even advise the patient to discontinue the study medication and/or hospital visits. I wonder whether it would be opportune to include in relevant protocols express recommendations to the investigators on how to approach the family doctors.

Due to limitations which will be discussed later, the objectives of an extensive clinical trial should be very clearly defined, because the organizational efforts involved in setting it up can vary considerably according to its aims.

If the drug is distributed to a large number of GPs with the request that they merely report their overall clinical impression, even according to a standardized procedure, the return on all this effort will only be information on the drug's general acceptability and tolerability.

When a protocol with more specific admission and evaluation criteria is provided, fresh estimates of the drug's activity in relation to given criteria (for example, sex, age or occupation) will be obtained.

If comparisons with alternative treatments or between different dosage schedules are set up, information similar to that gathered by a controlled clinical trial will be acquired, with possible limitations in the inferences which can be drawn.

General practitioners could also carry out a simplified form of "active" drug surveillance, although there are obvious difficulties in performing re-challenges and thus establishing a reliable cause–effect relationship.

How should a trial be carried out in general practice?

Difficulties and practical problems

At medical school, very little attention is given to the problems relating to the clinical evaluation of drugs. The doctor usually graduates with the uncritical conviction that the new medicines presented to him by drug firm representatives have been fully characterized.

Social medicine does not consider the scientific approach to medical practice. The doctor is often seen as an official, and he is required to deal with a lot of red tape, which is very time-consuming and not very intellectually rewarding. This adds to a GP's professional routine and makes him a very busy man indeed. He hates any additional work, like filling in special forms or keeping records which he may not consider strictly necessary for that particular patient.

Usually, during the time allotted to the study, any one doctor treats a limited number of patients with a given disease. Only occasionally is it possible to obtain a therapeutic assessment from him which is not a mere clinical impression, even if simple criteria are chosen, like blood pressure or body weight. On the other hand the simple pooling of data coming from different doctors and collected from heterogeneous groups of patients creates interpretation difficulties.

Methodological problems

In a clinical trial involving many doctors the use of placebo should be discouraged. In fact, it is illegal to include placebos in commercial presentations of drugs and, on the other hand, the use of a placebo, even in a special presentation, presents the average general practitioner whose training in clinical pharmacology is usually rather scanty with a problem of conscience. It is also true that placebo-controlled studies should have been performed in earlier phases, and need not be repeated unnecessarily. Therefore if a control group is planned, these subjects should be given a reference drug or different doses of the study drug.

When the planned trial is comparative, the issue of randomization arises. Experience has shown that the random allocation of treatments among a doctor's practice is fraught with problems: the very concept of randomization is foreign to the general practitioner. I believe that no clinical monitor would happily give the task of following the randomization list to any practising doctor.

A valid solution could be to consider the doctor rather than the patient as an experimental unit, randomly assigning to each participating physician only one of the treatment modes (say a dose, a reference drug), balancing the allocation according to any potential response-influencing factors (for example geographical location, urban/rural areas, young/old doctors, etc.). Analysis of data can be performed on the "global" response from the single doctors, considering, for instance, "favourable" a doctor who obtained a favourable response in the majority of his patients. The selection of the percentages which assess a doctor as "favourable" or "unfavourable" should obviously be established in advance by the protocol. A more traditional analysis on patient data can also be performed.

In an extensive clinical trial (Canti and Lucchelli 1971) we studied different dosage schedules of a drug indicated in the treatment of venous disorders, using symptomatic criteria for the evaluation of the response. Four hundred and thirty-three practising doctors from all the Italian regions treated 7,588 patients. A dose-response curve was obtained, which showed clearly that the highest dose did not give a better response than the one immediately preceding (Fig. 1), but yielded instead a larger number of side effects. Analysis on the doctors as experimental units gave similar results to those obtained when the patients were considered as experimental units.

It is well known that providing the patients with detailed instructions about a prescribed drug improves compliance and consequently the sensitivity of a trial (Haines 1976, Morris and Halperin 1979). We demonstrated that the set of instructions given to general practitioners can condition performance in carrying out a clinical trial (Selvini 1976, Basagni et al. 1977). A sample of practising doctors representative of the Milan area was divided at random into two comparable subgroups, each unaware of the other

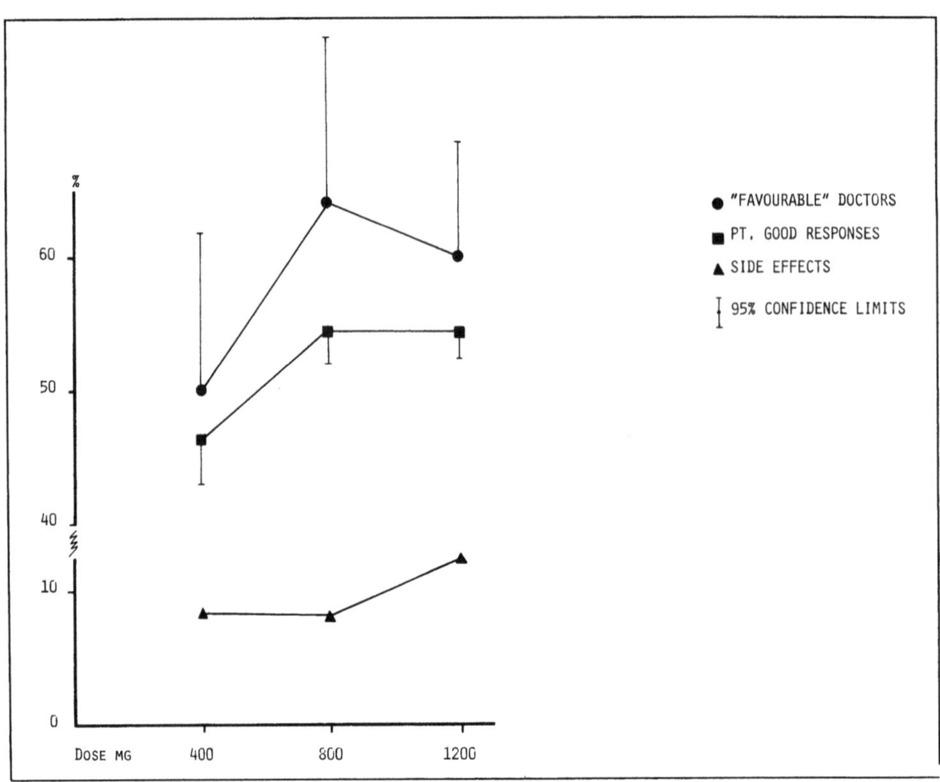

Fig. 1. Dose-response curves in a large-scale trial in general practice (from Canti and Lucchelli (2), mod. See text).

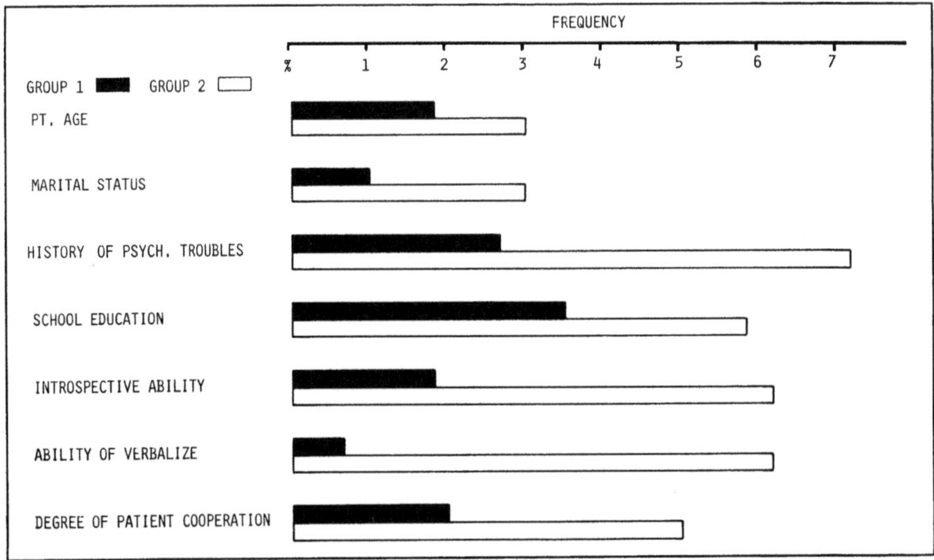

Fig. 2. Accuracy of doctors as measured by the frequency of lacking answers in a record form (from Basagni et al. (1)).

54

group. They were invited to carry out a trial on the treatment of patients with minor depressive illness. The first group was introduced to the problem of depression by an internist versed in Balint's techniques, who stressed the advisability and utility of a psychological approach to the patient, and gave reading suggestions and advice. The study was presented to the other group in the conventional way as a therapeutic trial on a psychoactive drug. The doctors of the first group treated more patients, gave more accurate responses and recorded more significant symptoms than the doctors of the second group (Fig. 2). The way the doctors are instructed to perform a trial should therefore be considered in any trial in general practice.

Organizational problems

An extensive trial can easily include hundreds of doctors and thousands of patients. The organization problems are enormous, including preparation and presentation of the protocol, collection and monitoring of case record forms, data transfer to computers and data analysis.
In the preparation of the protocol, at the risk of sacrificing sensitivity in the interests of homogeneity, the rule of thumb is simplicity and clarity: clarity in the objectives – few simple questions to obtain accurate replies; clarity in the admission and evaluation criteria – few simple variables which are easy to record with unequivocal meaning, so that valid generalizations may be drawn.
Monitoring can present difficulties; protocols and material may have to be distributed by the drug company representatives, who should also monitor the study. Training and motivation of this force are of paramount importance.

Conclusive remarks

Methodological and procedural limitations of extensive clinical trials often make a compromise necessary between what is theoretically desirable and what is practically feasible. Careful checks must be made of results to give reasonable confidence in their reliability.
Despite these operational limitations, the rationale for extensive clinical trials conducted on a newly released drug is still valid. It can yield valuable information. It can be a means of allowing the family doctor to combine science and art in the practice of medicine. It answers to needs of scientific knowledge and professional ethics. It is finally an important educational tool for the general practitioner, so often distracted by a routine workload, since a doctor who knows personally and responsibly how to study a drug is a better doctor than one who simply follows the usage recommendations.

References

1. Basagni M, Baroni L, Lucchelli PE (1977) Diagnostic policies of minor depressive illness by two differently trained groups of general practitioners. Int J Clin Pharmacol 15:474–476
2. Canti D, Lucchelli PE (1971) Effects of Glyvenol in relation to the dosage schedule employed (results of a large-scale trial in general practice). In: Kappert A (ed) Current aspects of chronic venous insufficiency. Ciba Geigy, Basel, p 186–200

3. Haines RB (1976) Strategies for improving compliances: a methodologic analysis and review. In: Sackett DL and Haines RB (eds) Compliance with Therapeutic Regimens. The Johns Hopkins University Press, Baltimore London, p 69–82
4. Lasagna L. This volume, P 45–49
5. Morris LA, Halperin JA (1979) Effects of written drug information on patient knowledge and compliance: a literature review. Am J Public Health 69:47–52
6. Selvini A (1976) Depression: a psychoterapeutic approach. In: Cassano GB, Lucchelli PE (eds) Psychosomatics and depression in general practice. Pozzi, Roma, p 10–17
7. Wheatley D (1973) Clinical Evaluation and Use of Drugs in General Practice. In: Jouhar AJ, Grayson MF (eds) International Aspects of Drug Evaluation and Usage. Churchill Livingstone, Edinburgh London, p 301–308

Author's address:
Paolo E. Lucchelli M.D.
Midy SpA, Sanofi Group
Via Piranesi 38
I-20137 Milano
Italy

Discussion

LUCCHELLI:
The discussion concerned the feasibility of having general practitioners conduct phase II studies. The speaker felt that practitioners should not be responsible for such trials but could play an important role in supporting phase II studies conducted by hospital physicians in ambulatory patients.

Clinical trials and chronic diseases

G. Fülgraff

A paradigm can be briefly described as the convention with which a majority of scientists in a certain field and at a given time see and define "reality". It is a widely and implicitly accepted framework, or system of reference, and the natural mode and the obviously reasonable way to look at things and to approach problems and procedures. Once established, it exerts a kind of unconscious psychic influence and steering power upon its adherents, who usually consider it a waste of time to question its premises but rather tend to interpret even opposing results as proof positive for the paradigm (Kuhn 1972).

The paradigm of scientific and practical medicine grew up during the 19th century. It was firmly established by its success as it became possible to discern specific external causes for specific diseases. Therefore the goal was to find the "cause" of a disease, to eliminate it, and to repair defects. This approach was successful with acute diseases and particularly with those generated by microorganisms, and hence it tended to reinforce itself: to find and eliminate specific causes.

Nowadays we have come to realize that chronic and irreversible diseases dominate, the courses of which are influenced also by biographical and psychic factors. But medicine remains focussed on the treatment of acute events occurring during the course of a chronic disease and on parameters, symptoms, and syndroms capable of being easily described, defined, and generalized. In this respect the paradigm demonstrates again and again its strength in explaining and prognosticating, but fails, however, when it comes to explaining or prognosticating the disease itself.

In order to make up for theoretical deficits, practical medicine, regardless of scientific scruples, falls back on the first principle of medical pragmatics: who cures, is right, whereby "practical medical experience" proves to be "not identical with scientific experience in medicine" (Buchborn 1983). The art of medicine therefore either escapes total scientific formalization or gives up both its usefulness and its possibilities. But this is just what would happen if medical theory and teaching insisted on passing on only those experiences which can be generalized and repeated at any time.

Clinical pharmacology and scientific drug research have been woven into this dichotomy of paradigm and theoretical deficit since the very beginning. In this context let me quote Paul Martini (1932), the founder of modern scientific clinical drug research, who wrote in the preface of the first edition of his "Methods of Therapeutic Investigation" in 1932: "The ultimate aim of scientific methods is the definitely determined experiment, the pure case. Only this and nothing else asks always the same question of nature to which nature always gives the same answer by virtue of its lawfulness and causality: A single clear-cut experiment, therefore, is of higher importance than any accumulation

---

Dedicated to Professor Dieter Palm on the occasion of his 60th birthday

of facts." With the latter, Martini refers to Poincaré, who said: "Science is made of facts as a house is made of bricks, but an accumulation of facts is no more a science than a heap of bricks is a house." And Martini continues: "Medicine has at least to approach exact induction." Apart from the fact that the term "exact induction" would drive any epistemologist to despair, what happens when nature does not behave as lawfully and causally as is implicated in the statement and as Martini obviously supposed in 1932? I certainly do not want to judge Martini by these phrases, a man who merits high esteem for his approach – at the time new and original – to a scientific evaluation of drugs; but it is worthwhile to remember what kind of untenable ideas – at least untenable in to-day's view – have been midwife at the birth of clinical drug research – and are still widely adhered to.

The methodology of clinical drug research is, on the one hand, related to the paradigm of medicine and, on the other hand, forms and influences pharmacotherapy in medical practice. Teachers and textbooks of pharmacotherapy and of clinical medicine stress the importance of an *individual* treatment of the *individual* patient, the *individual* choice of a drug, its form, dose, and dosage intervals; no one patient resembles the next; the treatment must be adapted to the patient and *his* disease. But how can this be done, seeing that in the scientific evaluation of drugs, from which practical application is derived, great efforts are exerted in dissolving the individualities of patients into groups; in comparing parameters or groups of parameter-bearers that have been randomized, stratified, etc.? Procrustes as the patron-saint of clinical trialists?

What is actually the scientific basis of deriving statements on an individualized therapeutic treatment from generalized statistical data on groups of parameter-bearers? The practice is known, but what are the theoretical grounds it is based upon? Is it not high time to consider and develop methods of gathering experiences on therapeutics and to make them intersubjectively communicable without binding individual patients into collective packages?

In the book "Un Dramma Borghese" by the Italian writer Guido Morselli (1978) a rheumatic patient on becoming aware once again of his sensations and reactions, reflects as follows: "This is, of course, a description which I would never give to a physician, not even to the physician I trust. Medicine tends to categorize and so does even the most modest practitioner; medicine distrusts the individual, i.e. the concrete experience." The patient is obviously afraid of losing the experience of his own personal illness, i.e. to lose this eventually last private corner, where individuality can still express itself. "To my mind, the singularity of a disease is different from what is called statistical deviation of an otherwise classifiable phenomenon", writes the physiologist and doyen of German social medicine Hans Schaefer in objecting to all attempts of categorizing individual experiences of being sick – the single casus – into a typus of sickness. "A thus standardized therapy must necessarily remain symptomatic because it does by definition not reach the essence of the disease" (Schaefer 1983). But if this is a consequence of the paradigm and of our methodology to investigate and to evaluate therapeutics, should we then not call into question our methods, thus enabling us to find really new principles? Is it a prerequisite for successful efforts to find drugs or therapeutic strategies for chronic diseases, to reconsider our understanding of these diseases? These questions can neither be easily answered nor put aside, since it remains a fact that there are no or very few other than symptomatically oriented drugs available for chronic diseases.

In the preface to the second edition of his "Methodology of Clinical-Therapeutic Research" Martini wrote in 1945: "Whoever declares a particular methodology of clinical therapeutic research to be necessary, obviously takes simple practical medical experience as not being sufficient" (1945). Experience, and how it is acquired, is a common problem of epistemology since Aristotle; and many and not the least minds of the medical profession reflect and dispute from time to time on the essence of practical medical experience. Hence, "simple" practical medical experience is not nearly as simple as it sounds, but what Martini and with him and following him many others wanted and still want, is to formalize decision-making processes and by these means make them "objective". Being sceptical if this formalization is in a strict sense possible, we must ask if – consequently carried out and being successful – it is desirable. It would mean, after all, substituting reality with a model which would have to be the more reductionist the more complex reality is, until finally only those sectors of reality would be perceived which occur in the model and the model would become a mould for the real world. Practical medical experience would thus not be gathered any more, activity and treatment being oriented toward the model and not toward real life.

How can this development be avoided? How can the reference to the reality of the individual sick person be reintegrated into clinical drug research? And how can the importance of a physician's empathy, and comprehensive experience, of the hermeneutic process and understanding be included, and investigations and assessments on therapeutics be based upon less formal grounds?

"The more a disease is modified or even caused not by standardizable environmental influences but rather by psychic factors, the more the physician is left alone by the results of clinical observational studies and even more of controlled and randomized trials" (Schaefer 1983), among other reasons because of the lack of individual biographical determinants of the disease not only in the studies but also in the underlying model. The course of chronic diseases is perhaps less regular and determined than the model implies. And might we not connect this with the fact that clinical drug research has been of rather limited success so far in finding therapeutics for chronic diseases? This connection cannot be simply denied when we consider that clinical trials in chronic diseases are necessarily mainly focussed on acute events occurring during the course of the disease or – and this does not make it easier – on the non-occurrence of such events. The models are not yet sufficient for chronic diseases. And lifetime studies accompanying patients for years or decades are at best exceptionally possible. They would wear out generations of trialists until perhaps therapeutic strategies can be assessed which, by the time the study finished, had become out of fashion. But what kind of parameters are actually available to register, estimate, and evaluate sensations, feelings, happiness, quality of life, in short, the very subjective world of the chronically ill?

Franz Gross (1982), on the occasion of a short review of the studies on platelet function inhibiting drugs in secondary prevention of coronary heart disease made the statement: "None of the studies in which ASA has been compared with placebo has demonstrated an unequivocal result, i.e. a prevention of fatal or non-fatal secondary attacks after recovery from myocardial infarction." And: "The underlying results with acetylsalicylic acid do, in spite of the trend they show, not justify recommending the medicine generally." Ellen Weber (1984) has a similar judgement when writing: "Ultimately, the ... results rather than becoming reliable guides, have left the therapist more uncertain." She supposes a trend in favour of ASA, but states that, nevertheless, none of the critics would give up his interpretation that the proof of efficacy failed. This would demonstrate, "how little medical activities and also the expressed opinions need to follow the objectivated facts". I want to underline this statement as being characteristic for the acceptance of the results of studies: they are well accepted if they fit into the leading opinions; if not they are reinterpreted if feasible or criticized in a manner to make it possible to reject them for methodological reasons. In view of these results and the amounts of money and committment invested into these studies, Weber has raised some questions about their significance and eventual improvement, two of which I shall discuss.

She asks: "What portion of a population of patients must have a benefit from the positive result of a study to justify the study on ethical grounds?" A discussion of this question is all the more necessary, the greater the number of patients involved in a study must be to be able to demonstrate an advantage of a treatment compared to placebo. If, for instance, as done in the Lipid Research Clinics Coronary Primary Prevention Trial, one half of approximately 3,400 persons are treated with Cholestyramine for years, with the result that only 30 fatal myocardial infarctions occurred in the treated group compared to 38 in the control group, then it means that 8 out of approximately 1700 people treated had a benefit or that 1700 people have been treated for the benefit of 8. Of course, it sounds better to say that the risk of fatal heart attacks was lowered by 24% (over-all mortality not being different). In many studies on primary or secondary prevention, huge numbers of patients have been treated whereas the expected benefit concerned only a few people and, hence, a very small proportion. Any difference, however miniscule, can be made to appear "statistically significant" with enough perseverance, enough money, and huge patient populations; but what, then, is the meaning? The consequence for medical practice, the unscreened prescription to large numbers of patients exposes all these persons to the risk of adverse reactions to the applied drugs, whereas very few can enjoy the benefit – besides the pharmaceutical companies involved. Thereby the question of ethics is raised not only for the clinical trials themselves but also for translation into medical practice. One can agree with M. F. Oliver who wrote (1984): "The risk of correcting risks by drugs may be greater than the uncorrected risk."

A second statment by Weber (1984) is that "the systematic search for subgroups with different pathomechanisms but similar symptoms has been greatly neglected". The above mentioned fact, that in many particularly extensive studies only a few of the many patients treated derived benefit, showed that the patient population was heterogeneous in spite of comparable qualifying symptomatology. I would therefore rather invest more resources in exploring the diseases and the differences in their development in order to be able to screen and to discriminate a patient population into subgroups, however small, with homogeneous etiology and pathogenetic factors, so that all patients of a subgroup can benefit from treatment of the same kind; this would mean giving priority to the *casus* instead of the *typus*. Doubtless far fewer patients would be needed for a meaningful study; on the other hand, the market for the product in question would be substantially smaller. There perhaps lies a possible reason why this kind of research has been somehow forced into the shadows of the gigantic studies. For, as many examples of such studies show, neither substantial influence on the opinion of previously convinced scientists – i.e. an influence on the prevailing paradigms – nor an unequivocally accepted improvement in the care for patients, nor answers for the

60

questions of medical practice can be expected; at best we can expect a transient enlargement of a specific portion of the pharmaceutical market. I do not consider the money spent for that in the long run a good investment.

Several epidemiological follow-up studies have yielded the conclusion that persons with mild or borderline hypertension can develop very differently: their blood pressure can return to normal, it can remain in the borderline range, or rise, with all the complications known to the hypertension disease. It would be of substantial advantage to these patients if better tools and criteria were available to recognize and to prognosticate those with a higher probability of future hypertension and to observe and eventually treat them instead of proposing drug treatment for all patients with mild hypertension. "Unless we can better define those people with mild hypertension who will benefit most from therapy (and those who will come to no harm if left untreated) the community benefit would be bought at the expense of many previously symptom-free individuals who would experience drug side-effects and derive no benefit", says the analysis of the joint World Health Organisation/International Society of Hypertension Mild Hypertension Liaison Committee (of which F. Gross was a member) (1982). An indiscriminate prophylactic pharmacotherapy of mild hypertension would affect a considerable proportion (15–20%) of the adult population in industrialized countries, exposing them to the adverse reactions of the drugs. As far as community medicine is concerned, there are also no arguments in favour of an indiscriminate drug therapy (Borgers 1982, Rose 1981).

The situation is comparable to that of the treatment of myocardial infarction or to that of secondary prevention. Sullivan (1979) wrote in a short comment to a study: "In view of these results, how is the patient with an acute myocardial infarction best managed? Arguments can be made for giving all patients prophylactic lidocaine to prevent subsequent ventricular fibrillation. Persuasive arguments can be made for the benefits of anticoagulant therapy. Evidence can be found to support the treatment of all patients with beta-adrenergic-receptor blocking compounds during the convalescent phase of acute anterior myocardial infarction. There is reason to consider using sulfinpyrazone during the first year after infarction to prevent sudden death. Now there is reason to consider the use of streptokinase during the acute phase of myocardial infarction. Should all patients receive the therapeutic mélange outlined above?... Each component of therapy has potential dangers and should be used only after individual judgements are made about individual patients."

But how can a physician facing his patient make this "individual judgement", when the clinical pharmacology only yields studies with an indiscriminate therapy for all patients with certain symptoms? Examples are known of studies, which, in spite of the huge number of patients, did not have the expected positive results; subsequent and ex post analyses of subgroups demonstrated, however, a benefit for a defined subgroup of patients with more specific risks.

Would it not be more reasonable to develop criteria to discern those patients – i.e. the more homogeneous subgroup – for whom a specific therapy is more suitable, than to carry out mass studies? Whatever the result of such studies might be – and with a study population of appropriately high size it will rarely fail to yield something "significant", whatever this means – it cannot be transferred into the therapeutic practice of a responsibly acting physician; the specific benefits for certain defined patients are masked and diluted in an unspecific crowd.

Results of clinical studies can hardly call into question the prevailing paradigms, but, on the other hand, studies are more readily accepted the better they fit into a predominant scientific consensus. As Mitchell wrote (1981) "We must remember the reluctance of editors to accept and of authors to offer negative trial results; in any condition reports of positive associations always outnumber valid but unexciting negative reports." And Weber states that "even the non-proven view is accepted, if it leads to a prescription."

Even the very expensive US Multiple Risk Factor Intervention Trial could not change anybody's conviction. Advocates and sceptics of this kind of intervention find their views corroborated and will certainly continue to argue with each other using the same results, whereby the advocates have the advantage of swimming in the paradigm. The most surprising result of the MRFIT-study was, however, that the drug treatment of mild hypertension for a subgroup of men with abnormal baseline electrocardiograms was not only of no benefit but actually rather harmful (MRFIT Research Group 1982; Kaplan 1983). It is therefore urgent to reassess the recommendations for drug treatment of mild hypertension.

How else than with paradigmatic partial blindness can it, for example, be explained, when it has been written in a survey on hypertension intervention trials, that those trials which failed to demonstrate an advantage of intervention had obviously been wrongly designed, since with a correct methodological approach they should have had positive results? Or what can a reader learn, when in a study on treatment of hypertension four drugs were investigated as possible third agent in combination with a beta-adrenergic-blocking agent and a diuretic with the result that two of the drugs were suited and the other two not, and when the authors write, that these came off badly only because their peculiarities had not been sufficiently considered in the protocol? Or when the superiority of surgical treatment of coronary heart disease has been demonstrated by comparing its recent results with former studies on drug-treated patients, thus neglecting the progress in drug therapy, whereas the CASS trial (1984) showed that using comparable standards there are no differences in mortality or occurrence of reinfarction? Or when one could read in a well respected German medical journal about a certain unconventional therapeutic procedure: "This method is still contested albeit in the meanwhile well-substantiated by a series of trials and case studies." Of what use, therefore, are such trials, when they do not happen to fit into the prevailing opinion?

I would like to sum up this short excursion into some theoretical problems of clinical drug research in three appeals:

- Often, practical medicine does not receive answers to the questions which it asks of scientific clinical drug research, but rather to questions which it does not ask and which can be suitably answered with the available methodology. Instead of requesting that from medical practice other – the right – questions be asked, efforts should be undertaken to further develop the methodology to be able to answer the questions which are really asked.

- The individuality of patients, the quality of life of the chronically diseased and the hermeneutic approach to disease and the way it is coped with should be integrated into the design of clinical drug research to prevent a gap between research and medical practice.

- Therapeutic research in general and drug research in particular should be careful not to miss the possible appearance on the scene of practical medicine of a new paradigm, of a new understanding of man, his health and disease.

References

1. Borgers D (1982) Risikofaktorenmedizin und Primärprävention beim milden Bluthochdruck. Münch Med Wochenschr 124:655–659
2. Buchborn E (1983) Erfahrung in der Medizin (Editorial). Münch Med Wochenschr 125:185–186
3. CASS Principal Investigators and their Associates (1984) Myocardial infarction and mortality in the Coronary Artery Surgery Study (CASS) randomized trial. New Engl J Med 310:750–758
4. Gross F (1982) Infarktprophylaxe und Verhütung des plötzlichen Herztodes? (Editorial). Münch Med Wochenschr 124:435–436
5. Kaplan NM (1983) New approaches to the therapy of mild hypertension. Am J Cardiol 51:621–627
6. Kuhn TS (1972) Die Struktur wissenschaftlicher Revolutionen. Suhrkamp, Frankfurt am Main
7. Martini P (1932) Methodenlehre der therapeutischen Untersuchung. Springer, Berlin
8. Martini P (1945) Methodenlehre der therapeutisch-klinischen Forschung. Springer, Berlin
9. Mitchell JRA (1981) Timolol after myocardial infarction: an answer or a new set of questions? Br Med J 282:1565–1570
10. Morselli G (1978) Un Dramma Borghese. Adelphi Edizioni, Milano
11. Multiple Risk Factor Intervention Trial (MRFIT) Research Group (1982) Multiple Risk Factor Intervention Trial. JAMA 248:1465–1477
12. Oliver MF (1982) Does control of risk factors prevent coronary heart disease? Br Med J 285:1065–1066
13. Rose G (1981) Strategy of prevention: Lessons for cardiovascular disease. Br Med J 282:1847–1851
14. Schaefer H (1983) Erfahrung nicht als Vorurteil ablehnen (Leserbrief). Münch Med Wochenschr 125 Nr 10:31–32
15. Sullivan JM (1979) Streptokinase and myocardial infarction. New Engl J Med 301:836–837
16. Weber E (1984) Problematik des Wirksamkeitsnachweises von Aggregationshemmern. Münch Med Wochenschr 126:336–340
17. World Health Organisation/International Society of Hypertension Mild Hypertension Liaison Committee (1982) Trials of the treatment of mild hypertension. Lancet I:149–156

Author's address:
Prof. Dr. G. Fülgraff
Clausewitzstraße 8
1000 Berlin 12
F.R.G.

Discussion

FÜLGRAFF:
The discussion emphasized the important difference between statistical significance and clinical relevance. With large-scale studies it is frequently possible to show statistically significant drug effects that are of no therapeutic interest to practitioners of medicine. On the other hand, even small increases in cure rates or in length of survival can be important if they are achieved in common diseases.

Alternatives to clinical trials in post-marketing research on drug effects

Olli S. Miettinen

Introduction

The speakers before me have addressed clinical experimentation as a basis for informed decisions about the use of drugs. My topic is alternatives to clinical trials, with special reference to drug evaluation after marketing (Phase IV). I shall deal with it from the vantage of a decade and a half of consultation work in this area, especially with the Drug Epidemiology Unit of Boston University School of Medicine.

Why post-marketing research?

For orientation, a few words about the need for post-marketing drug research may be in order.

That pre-marketing research provides an incomplete scientific foundation for optimal decision-making in the use of drugs is well known.

In the area of *efficacy* these deficiencies of Phase III research result from the following:

1. The drug use in those trials is generally quite *unrepresentative* of actual Phase IV use with respect to both the drug regimens themselves and the clinical situations in which they are used, to say nothing about the general failure of Phase III trials to study *various practically occurring regimens and clinical situations* per se.
2. Phase III trials generally address *absolute* efficacy, whereas in clinical decision-making the need usually is to know efficacy relative to available alternative drugs.
3. Those trials quite regularly address the *primary* effect of the drug, such as lowering of blood pressure, even when the actual purpose of using the drug is a presumed secondary effect, such as prevention of vascular complications of "hypertension".

We have recently reported on these deficiencies in the area of efficacy in quantitative terms, examining prescription drugs on the market in the United States (1).

With respect to *toxicity* the limited and unrepresentative nature of the regimens and clinical situations, and the focus on absolute effects, are analogous in their implications to those in the area of efficacy. Another limitation, specific to toxicity, is the *size* of Phase III trials: with only a few thousand patients typically involved, those trials do not provide assurance of safety in reference to rare but serious adverse reactions.

The deficiencies of the information from Phase III trials are often more obvious and striking in the context of indications that develop only after marketing. The dominant need for Phase IV research in this context relates to efficacy, of course, but new concerns about toxicity may arise from use of the drug on new types of patient.

Consultant, Drug Epidemiology Unit, Boston Unviersity School of Medicine

Why consider alternatives to clinical trials?

Beyond the *need* for Phase IV research on drug effects, my topic raises the orientational question of *why alternatives* to clinical trials need to be considered in Phase IV research. Clinical trials are, by definition, experimental studies. This means that, in such studies, patients are assigned to their particular treatment categories not on the basis of their presumed individual best interests but solely in the interest of learning about the effects of the treatment in general, the means to the latter end often being random allocation.
Naturally, experimental treatment allocation is consonant with clinical ethics only when there is true ambivalence about the choice of treatment, and this is somewhat of an exception today, especially in the context of Phase IV questions about the treatment of choice, albeit unjustifiably in many instances.
It is this ethical dilemma about experimental treatment allocation, justified or not, that poses the main obstacle for clinical trials in Phase IV research. An additional impediment for such studies is added logistical difficulty – even if the importance of this tends to be overemphasized.
While these problems with clinical trials in Phase IV obviously do call for the consideration for alternatives to them, it is to be understood that they represent, as a matter of logic, *nonexperimental* or quasi-experimental research – but not necessarily "post-marketing *surveillance*" (PMS). To be sure, surveillance is inherently nonexperimental, but the term properly refers to ongoing vigilance activities directed to potential adverse effects, excluding projects whose purpose is to quantify efficacy or known or suspected toxicity.

On what conditions are the alternatives valid?

Nonexperimental alternatives to clinical trials are, generally, subject to serious concerns about validity, and it is, thus, important to appreciate the conditions on which such studies are valid.
The essence of the validity conditions for nonexperimental research on drug effects flows from the fact that in nonexperimental experience with drug effects the counterpart of randomization is clinical decision. Such decision-making between the compared treatments can be essentially random. However, material nonrandomness can arise on account of differential indications or contraindications.
Thus, nonexperimental post-marketing research is valid if, and only if, differential indications and contraindications are either absent, unrelated to the outcome at issue, or measurable and thereby controllable.
These conditions are relevant primarily in studies in which the effect must be inferred by means of comparative statistical inference. If the effects can be determined on a patient-by-patient basis, the issue of confounding, whether by indication (2–4) or contraindication (4), is moot as long as the concern is with absolute effects only.

How commonly are the alternatives valid?

Given the potential problems of confounding by indication and/or contraindications, one wonders how commonly valid nonexperimental alternatives to clinical trials are available in Phase IV assessment of drug effects. An understanding of these issues requires that one distinguishes between efficacy and toxicity studies and, in the realm of the latter, between known or suspected toxicity on one side and unsuspected toxicity on the other.

In *efficacy* research the validity problem has to do with differential indications almost exclusively. Such differences in the severity of the indication are obviously quite common, especially in studies of absolute efficacy, and they relate to outcome criterion of efficacy studies as a matter of course – whenever the indication is rational. It is thus apparent a priori that confounding by indication is quite a common problem in efficacy research (2–4); and what is more, its control in nonexperimental studies tends to be hampered by the indication's subtlety and complexity (2). Our systematic review of recently marketed drugs (5) has averred this expectation and provided quantification of the frequency of occurrence of intractable difficulties.

When the concern is with *known or suspected toxicity,* the validity problem is conceptually analogous to that of efficacy studies, with contraindications the confounder in lieu of indication – but the problem is much lesser than in efficacy studies (2, 4). The basis for the difference is that while indication tends to be quite variable in its severity among patients, contraindications as a patient characteristic tend to be essentially invariant – by virtue of being absent in most instances. For this reason, confounding by contraindications is only occasionally an intractable problem in the study of known or suspected toxicity (4).

In post-marketing surveillance, concerned with the detection of unsuspected toxicity, there is no issue of contraindications by definition.

Strategies for post-marketing research

As it is apparent that there is a major need for post-marketing assessment of drug effects, and that such research is to address such drug-therapeutic practices as actually prevail in health care, there arise the questions of what *routine* data systems could be utilized or should be developed to meet the Phase IV research needs, and how the drug experience so captured should be scanned and analyzed.

Until now, attention to these matters has been focussed on the detection of unsuspected toxicity, with special reference to newly marketed drugs. Indeed, an extensive study and planning effort on this limited subject was carried out for the United States government several years ago (6) – though, alas, very little action has resulted from it.

The larger need is, however, to develop and implement a strategy to assess known and suspected toxicity as well, and efficacy in addition, all of these in the real-life environment of actual Phase IV experience. For, only the harvesting of this ultimately relevant experience in all relevant regards provides for realistic assessment of risk-benefit which, together with consideration of monetary costs, provides for truly enlightened use of drugs in the best interests of both patients and society.

References

1. Strom BL, Melmon KL, Miettinen OS (1985) Post-marketing studies of drug efficacy: why?
   Am J Med (in press)
2. Miettinen OS (1980) Efficacy of therapeutic practice: will epidemiology provide the answers?
   In: Melmon KL (ed) Drug Therapeutics: Concepts for Physicians. Elsevier-North Holland,
   New York, p 201–208
3. Strom BL, Miettinen OS, Melmon KL (1983) Post-marketing studies of drug efficacy: when
   must they be randomized? Clin Pharmacol Ther 34: 1–7
4. Miettinen OS (1983) The need for randomization in the study of intended effects. Statist Med
   2: 267–271
5. Strom BL, Miettinen OS, Melmon KL (1984) Post-marketing studies of drug efficacy: how? Am
   J Med 77: 703–708
6. IMS America Ltd, Health Care Research Group (1978) Final Report, Task A. An Experiment in Early Post-Marketing Surveillance of Drugs. DHEW/PHS/FDA, Rockville, Maryland

Author's address:
Olli S. Miettinen, M.D., Ph.D.
Professor of Epidemiology and Biostatistics
Professor of Medicine
Faculty of Medicine
McGill University
1020 Pine Avenue West
Montreal, Quebec H3A 1A2
Canada

Discussion

MIETTINEN:
The speaker was asked why he had not discussed spontaneous reporting of adverse drug reactions
in the context of postmarketing surveillance. It was pointed out that regulatory authorities are increasingly using information from spontaneous reporting systems as a basis for their decisions
about marketed drugs. Dr. Miettinen answered that in his view spontaneous reporting systems did
not qualify as research, addressed a relatively unimportant part of the drug safety problem and
need not concern us in decision making.

The future of long-term intervention
and prevention studies – methodological aspects

F. H. Epstein

Introduction

At a meeting in New York in 1968, Dr. Donald S. Fredrickson, the Director of the National Heart Institute in Bethesda at the time, gave an historic address with the title: "The Field Trial: some thoughts on the indispensable ordeal" (Fredrickson 1968). This was when the era of the large intervention studies started and trials like MRFIT were being planned. The sober words "indispensable" and "ordeal" which Fredrickson advisedly used, reflect the issue in a masterly fashion and stand, perhaps, in some contrast to the enthusiasm which characterized the creation and conduct of the subsequent studies. Presumably, without such a spirit, it would be impossible to carry out this kind of work at all. Today, 16 years later, much has been learned. Much has happened that is sobering but, on balance, there are grounds for satisfaction and hope for the future. It is, however, not the purpose of this review to attempt an evaluation of the preventive trials conducted during these years but to try, in a pragmatic and informal way, to discuss some of the methodological aspects of large intervention studies in the area of cardiovascular diseases. The review, not being systematic, will bypass some important issues like the need for monitoring and quantifying side-effects or for long-term follow-up of trial participants beyond the termination of the trial itself.

The need for large numbers

If it is the aim to show that certain measures will prevent disease or its recurrence (primary or secondary prevention), rather than merely the demonstration that risk factors for the disease can be reduced, the first problem to face is the need for large numbers of trial participants. It is no accident that there are so many more trials in the field of cardiovascular disease than, say, cancer, the reason being that the incidence of cancer, high though it is, is considerably lower than the incidence of, say, coronary heart disease. Coronary heart disease has a high incidence as far as chronic diseases go (in the region of 5 events per 1,000 per year among men) but not high enough to get away, as it were, with sample sizes under several thousands of persons over several years. This entails not only large costs but – and this is what causes much of the costs – a large staff to ensure participation and quality control, with all the attendant problems of organization. Actually, it is remarkable how well these problems of strategy and logistics can be solved, given the necessary support. All this is a long way from what Sir Austin Bradford Hill, truly the father of the concept of trials, originally had in mind when he first wrote about "Clinical Trials" over 30 years ago. In order to reduce sample sizes to manageable proportions, it is necessary to resort to high-risk groups for primary prevention or to secondary prevention trials, the price paid being the problem of extrapolating the results to the entire population or, respectively, to persons not yet ill. Whatever is important in ensuring the success of a trial is made more difficult if the sample must be large: attaining satisfactory differentials between treatment and reference groups, minimizing drop-outs and quality of data collection, all of which are needed, amongst other things, to achieve the desired statistical power.

Reference groups – double-blind designs

The choice of reference groups is a major concern. If it is a question whether a treatment is effective at all, a placebo will be used. In the case of a drug, this will imply double-blinding but if the treatment is, for example, a diet, a double-blind design is not generally feasible though it has been tried in the National Diet-Heart Feasibility Study. Increasingly, however, it is asked whether one treatment is better than another. This arises when it is considered unethical to have an untreated comparison group, as in the HDFP, LRC-CPPT and MRFIT trials in the United States (6, 7, 9). In this situation, it must be accepted in advance that the difference between the treated and reference groups may be relatively small so that greater numbers or a longer study are needed. There are no simple or generalizable answers to these questions. With the advent of "big epidemiology" and mass trials, new approaches had and will have to be designed.

Compliance and drop-outs

Various degrees of failure to adhere to the prescribed regimen or failure to continue participation in the trial for various reasons are facts of trial-life and they must be faced in the analysis and interpretation of the results. The issue has been well-stated in a recent book on biostatistics in medicine by Murphy (1982): "Once in the study, subjects may not merely die prematurely; they may be lured to a great distance by employment, politics or love; they may conceive a distaste for the investigator or the treatment and refuse to participate further; they may meddle illegally with the dosage which they are supposed to take, try supplementary medication, or pry into a blinding procedure. (I have had all these misfortunes overtake me in clinical studies.)"
What can be done if the drop-outs turn out to be different kinds of people in the experimental and reference groups? If those who comply better derive greater benefit from the treatment, is it justifiable to infer that this dose-response relationship strengthens the case for the existence of a causal relationship, even though there was no randomization? Once again, there is no over-all answer. For instance, if a placebo were given, it might be possible to demonstrate that the dose-response phenomenon was confined to the recipients of the active drug which would be strongly in support of a cause-and-effect relationship.

Relevance of the study population or the intervention used to the "real-life" situation

It happens frequently that the group which is eventually randomized into a trial is no longer representative of the entire universe of people who require care. This selection may be the result of ethical consideration, exclusion criteria or other reasons. An example is the recent Coronary Artery Surgery (CASS) Study which excluded patients with more severe disease, i.e. the very people who need treatment most (11). Relevance of the treatment used to the realities of daily medical care or, for that matter, daily living like eating habits, is another issue which usually comes to attention only after the termination of the trial when problems appear. The University Group Diabetes (UGDP) Study belongs in this category because the treatment used was fixed and not adapted to the condition of the patients at the time (15). The same was true to some extent with regard to thiazide dosage in the MRFIT study (1982) and may have contributed to the anomalous results in hypertensive persons with electrocardiographic changes (Stamler and Liu 1983). Prevention of these problems lies, as always, in recognizing them in advance. This does not necessarily ensure success since there is an inherent dilemma between the need for standardization and the need to adapt to changing circumstances.

Intervention in high-risk groups or the total population?

Among the lessons learned from coronary heart disease epidemiology is the realization that around half of the events of myocardial infarction and sudden death come from the fifth of the population at the highest risk in terms of the main risk factors whereas the remainder derive from the lower 4/5th of the multiple logistic risk function. This is itself implies that an effective strategy to prevent premature disease in the population must use a double strategy: (1) an intensive intervention programme for those at top risk and (2) a less intensive but still determined programme for the population at large, including young people. As mentioned already under the topic of "numbers", it is not possible to conduct a randomized, controlled trial in a whole population or sample because of the huge numbers required. The alternative is to use a high-risk group, as was done in MRFIT or part of the WHO European Trial (16), and to extrapolate the results to those at lower risk. While such extrapolations are often though not invariably justified scientifically, they may not satisfy those who have more rigid standards for accepting the validity of evidence. An example is the recently published LRC-CPPPT Study (7) in which the effectiveness of serum cholesterol and low-density lipoprotein lowering on reducing the risk of coronary heart disease amongst men with initially high levels was demonstrated. The question is whether serum lipid level lowering in the population at large would also prevent coronary heart disease. There are many arguments in favour of believing that it would but this view is not shared by those who would demand direct "proof".
It is becoming increasingly clear that it is very difficult to plan, design and conduct decisive randomized, large-scale trials to test the effectiveness of preventive measures in the community at large. Therefore, community studies – with test and reference areas – are being given increasing attention. The first of these was the Stanford Study (Farquhar 1978), soon followed by the North Karelia Project (3, 12). This is, however, not the place to compare and contrast randomized trials and community intervention studies.

Interpretation of results: sub-group analysis

Among the large number of questions arising in the course of analyzing the results of intervention trials, few if any are as troublesome as the matter of subgroup analysis.

The simplest is the purist approach which would not accept any analysis based on any other than the "intent-to-treat" group. If the trial turns out to be positive on this level, all is well and there is no further problem. Unfortunately, this is by no means the rule. On the contrary, it becomes more and more evident that trials concerned with primary or secondary prevention of chronic dieases as often as not turn up with results which are marginal or open to different interpretations. In this situation, it is tempting to engage, as it is sometimes called, in data dredging. This off-the-cuff derogatory attitude is unfortunate since there is nothing wrong in looking for internal inconsistencies within the totality of the data. If there are such inconsistencies which have a plausible explanation, it is entirely justified to conclude that the trial might have turned out more favourably if it had not been for these difficulties. On the other hand, it would be entirely wrong to claim on the basis of such considerations that the trial is positive when, in fact, it was negative in terms of the intention-to-treat analysis.

Two examples may be given. In beta-blocker trials, it appears that only patients with pre-existing cardiac insufficiency seem to derive benefit (5). Should this finding be disregarded just because the patients were not randomized in advance into those with and those without cardiac insufficiency? The MRFIT Study is frequently called "negative" and even quoted as indicating that primary prevention of coronary heart disease does not "work". In fact, the trial would have shown a positive result but for the group of hypertensives with electrocardiographic abnormalities in which those receiving "special care" had a higher incidence of disease than persons in the reference group (13). There are several possible explanations for this paradox finding, amongst others the curious phenomenon that in the reference group, hypertensives with abnormal electrocardiograms had a lower incidence than those with normal tracings which must have contributed to the anomalous result. To conclude from all this that the trial was, in fact, positive would be unwarranted and misleading in the extreme. However, the same should be said to those who call the result "negative" without any qualification.

A basic dilemma: how many people are treated "unnecessarily"?

It is frequently stated that primary prevention implies the need to treat a great number of people in order to protect a few. In other words, preventive care is said to be given to a large proportion of persons who would not become ill anyway and who will, therefore, be treated unnecessarily. To what extent is this true? The situation is quite different in the case of secondary prevention because, here, it is a matter of treating people who are already ill and asking for treatment. When, on the other hand, a physician recommends preventive care, he can only do so in good conscience if he feels even more convinced than in the case of curative care that the patients or, rather, patients-to-be are going to benefit. The problem will be illustrated by two examples, referring to the treatment of hypertension and hypercholesterinaemia in order to prevent cardiovascular complications.

For "middle-aged" hypertensive men, the risk of developing major cardiovascular complications over the years is very high, amounting to about 50 percent (Fig. 1). It is difficult to obtain this rate from the literature since the data are not published in a form that can be used. However, adding up roughly the several components of the entire category "cardiovascular diseases" from the book "The Framingham Study" (Dawber

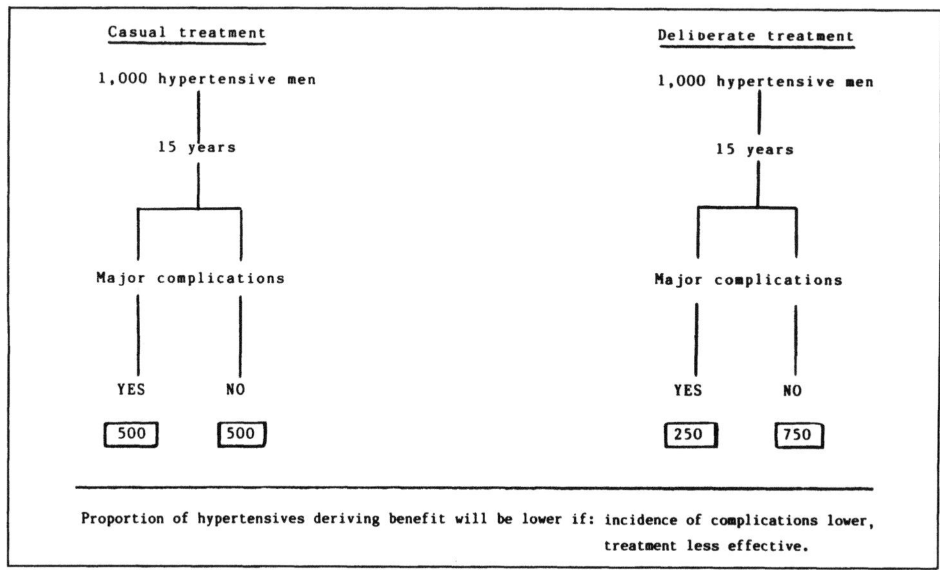

Fig. 1. Hypertension: How many people derive benefit from treatment?

1980) or using actual but unpublished data from the Framingham Study (personal communication from W. B. Kannel), it may be estimated that around half of all hypertensive men develop one or the other major cardiovascular complications within 15 years. This estimate applies to middle-aged men, the risk for women being between 40–50% lower. The complications included are coronary heart disease, stroke, cardiac failure and intermittent claudication. Let it be assumed that preventive treatment can lower the risk by 50 percent. This is within the range of effectiveness of the only large, placebo-controlled study reported so far – the Australian trial (8). On that assumption, 250 events will have been prevented, leaving 750 instead of 500 men free of complications within the time period. How many men were, so to speak, treated "unnecessarily"? On the face of it, the answer is 500 men because they would have remained without overt disease manifestations. In other words, half of the 1,000 men with hypertension have to be treated "unnecessarily" in order to protect a quarter of them. There is, however, another way to look at the numbers. In the group treated deliberately, it may be said that one in three hypertensives (250 out of 750), remaining free of complications, would have become ill without adequate therapy. A chance of 1 : 3 represents a very high individual risk. From the population point of view, protecting 250 out of a thousand men at the price of treating twice as many (500), as it were, unnecessarily is not an unreasonable price to pay. It lies in the nature of prevention that more people must be treated prophylactically than will derive benefit. This is tacitly accepted in the case of immunizations but the situation there is obviously quite different since a few injections cannot be compared to drug treatment with its side-effects, continued over years. The solution would lie in being able to prevent and treat hypertension by non-pharmacological and safe means. The calculations just made turn out less favourably if the incidence of complications is lower or treatment is less effective. There is, at this time, no clear-cut or simple answer to these problems, until effective methods for the

73

Table 1. How many persons derive benefit from preventive treatment? Example: *LRC-CPPT* trial. Men aged 35–59 years (av. 48 years)

	Duration of trial 7.4 years		Estimated probability of developing CHD between ages of 30 and 60 years*			
			Conservative		Realistic	
	Placebo	Drug**	Placebo	Drug	Placebo	Drug
CHD***	100	80	400	200	500	250
No CHD	900	920	600	800	500	750
Total	1 000	1 000	1 000	1 000	1 000	1 000

   * Based on N. J. Stone, R. I. Levy, D. S. Fredrickson, D. S. and J. Verter »Coronary Artery Disease in 116 Kindred with Familial Type II Hyperlipoproteinemia«, Circulation 49: 476–788, 1974 (Appendix II, Table 2).

  ** Drug: Cholestyramine

*** CHD: myocardial infarction or cardiac death

identification of low-risk hypertensives are found so that only those at high risk need to be treated.

Interestingly enough, the data from the recently completed Lipid Research Clinics – Coronary Primary Prevention Trial (LRC-CPPT) lead to conclusions similar to those just reached (Table 1). The randomized trial (7), including 3,806 middle-aged men with hypercholesterinaemia, was aimed at reducing the incidence of coronary heart disease through serum cholesterol and low-density lipoprotein lowering, comparing a group receiving the drug cholestyramine and a diet with a group receiving dietary treatment only. The actual results, calculated per thousand men, are shown in the left-hand panel, indicating that the incidence in the group receiving placebo and diet was about 10% over the 7.4 years of the trial. Under active treatment with cholestyramine, the incidence decreased 20%, to 80/1,000, which was statistically significant. However, the true risk of coronary heart disease between the ages of 30 and 60 years is probably much higher than the LRC-CPPT trial would suggest at first glance, being at least 40% and more likely 50%, as shown in the table. This estimate is derived from the comprehensive study of coronary heart disease in hyperlipoproteinaemia (14) and also the trial itself, quadrupling the 7.4 year incidence to cover 30 years. In addition, the true effect of treatment is greater than the trial average suggests because men who took the full dose of the drug had a lowering of risk, not of 20 but 50%. Taking the "realistic" estimated probability of developing coronary heart disease, the figures become identical with those used in the hypertension model, leading to the same inferences.

"Is your trial really necessary?"

The question is paraphrased from a poster which was seen in Britain everywhere during the Second World War: "Is your journey really necessary?". This question was intended to make people think twice before deciding to make a journey since travelling impeded the War effort in several ways. Before embarking on a trial, it must be asked whether it is really necessary. Looking back on the last 10 or 20 years, one may wonder if the large or very large trials to test whether or to what degree coronary heart disease and related disorders could be delayed by preventive treatment using drugs or changes in life-style were worth-while. The over-all answer is probably affirmative, in the sense that these were "indispensable ordeals" which had to be set up and carried through. Much has been learned and much of it has been encouraging. At the same time, it is also true that the results have been, on the whole, less decisive than had been hoped. Instead of providing "proof", the data, even if positive, have frequently been open to controversial interpretations. If the hope was that risk could be halved, the observed order of magnitude was usually though not always around 20–25%. A good deal of all this is no doubt due to "too little having been done too late" (2) since chronic diseases like atherosclerosis develop slowly over many years and it may be unreasonable to expect dramatic results when preventive efforts are started in middle-age. In view of this, what has been achieved is all the more remarkable.

Where do we go from here? As far as preventive treatment with pharmacological agents is concerned, whether for primary or secondary prevention, the categorical answer is that there is no alternative to controlled trials, with monitoring of side-effects and long-term follow-up. When a major emphasis of the preventive effort is on changes in life-style, community projects with reference communities, along the pattern of the Stanford or North Karelia Studies (3, 12), are the likely first choice for the future. Doing randomized trials like MRFIT in this area is very difficult, very expensive, uses artificial settings for the intervention methods and takes no advantage of community interactions which facilitate participation. Effective prevention is in all likelihood, as should have been learned, more than only "risk-factor engineering", important though it is. If there is a specific question to be answered, it must be asked first whether a trial would contribute to providing it. Even if it would, a trial may not be feasible or likely to be decisive. Much has been learned in recent years about estimating what can and cannot be expected from trials, whether based on randomized individuals or the community, to what extent intervention methods can be effectively instituted and how much yield can be reasonably expected. This should stand future planning in good stead.

Summary

Some methodological aspects of large-scale intervention studies, especially in the field of cardio-vascular diseases are discussed in terms of the number of participants required, the choice of reference groups, double-blind design, compliance and drop-outs, relationships between the study population and the universe at large, trials in high-risk groups as opposed to trials in the general population, community intervention studies, the problems of sub-group analysis and, particularly, the question deriving from the results of trials, how many persons must be treated "unnecessarily" in order to protect a relative minority from clinical disease. It is concluded that the proportion of those who will receive "unnecessary" treatment is, in general, not unreasonably high, that prevention by pharmaceutical measures requires testing by means of preventive trials while prevention through changes in life style is tested most effectively by means of community studies.

References

1. Dawber TR (1980) The Framingham Study. The Epidemiology of Atherosclerotic Disease. Harvard University Press, Cambridge and London
2. Epstein FH (1977) Preventive trials and the "diet-heart" question: wait for results or act now? Atherosclerosis 26:515–523
3. Farquhar JW (1978) The community-based model of life-style intervention trials. Am J Epidemiol 108:103–111
4. Fredrickson DS (1968) The field trial: some thoughts on the indispensable ordeal. Bull NY Acad Med 44:985–993
5. Furberg CD (1984) personal communication
6. Hypertension and Detection Follow-up Program Cooperative Group (1979) Five- year findings of the hypertension and detection follow-up program. JAMA 242:2562–2571
7. Lipid Research Clinics Program (1984) Reduction in incidence of coronary heart disease. JAMA 251:351–364
8. Management Committee (1980) The Australian therapeutic trial in mild hypertension. Lancet I:1261–1267
9. Multiple Risk Factor Intervention Trial Research Group (1982): Multiple risk factor intervention trial. JAMA 248:1465–1477
10. Murphy EA (1982) Biostatistics in Medicine. Baltimore. The Johns Hopkins University Press
11. Myocardial infarction and mortality in the coronary artery surgery study (CASS) randomized trial (1984) New Engl J Med 310:750–758
12. North Karelia Project (1981) Community Control of Cardiovascular Diseases. Copenhagen, Regional Office for Europe, World Health Organization.
13. Stamler J and Liu K (1983) The benefits of prevention. In: Prevention of Coronary Heart Disease (NM Kaplan and J Stamler eds) Philadelphia, WB Saunders Co, pp 188–207
14. Stone NJ et al (1974) Coronary artery disease in 116 kindreds with familial type II hyperlipoproteinemia. Circulation 49II:476–488
15. University Group Diabetes Program (1970) A study of the effects of hypoglycemic agents on vascular complications. Diabetes [Suppl 2] 19:7477–7830
16. World Health Organization European Collaborative Group (1983) Multifactorial trial in the prevention of coronary heart disease: Mortality and incidence results. Europ Heart J 4:141–147

Author's address:
Frederick H. Epstein, M.D.
Lindenstraße 37
CH-8008 Zürich
Switzerland

Discussion

EPSTEIN:
In the discussion of this paper full agreement was apparent on the need for identification of patients who are at special risk even within high risk groups. This consideration applies both to prevention studies and to intervention with specific patients. There is also a need to learn more about the less well known risk factors such as psychological characteristics, social class and genetic markers.

Lessons for the future from long-term studies with beta blockers and hypolipidaemic agents

J. D. Fitzgerald

Introduction

Most large pharmaceutical companies have devoted a significant proportion of their research investment to the discovery of new ways of combating cardiovascular disease. This is because coronary artery and cerebral vascular disease are major causes of morbidity and mortality in the Western World. The approach favoured in the Pharmaceuticals Divison of Imperial Chemical Industries PLC in the late 1950s was firstly to reduce, or even reverse, the progression of the atherosclerotic process in coronary artery disease by reducing serum cholesterol. This research resulted in the discovery of clofibrate ('Atromid')* by Mr. Thorp, which has become the reference hypolipidaemic agent (Thorp 1963). The second approach was to improve the metabolic status of the ischaemic myocardium by reducing the increase in cardiac work due to sympathetic stimulation by antagonising the action of noradrenaline on cardiac adrenoceptors. Such antagonists are now referred to as beta blockers and the reference compound is propranolol ('Inderal')* (Black 1967 & Fitzgerald 1972). During the succeeding 25 years innumerable studies have been carried out with these and other entities with a similar mode of action in order to determine their effect on morbidity and mortality in cardiovascular disease. In this review I wish to dwell upon the lessons for the future from such studies, but in order to derive such lessons it is necessary to summarize the trials results.

Studies with beta blockers

The results of all published trials designed to evaluate the effects of beta blockade on morbidity and mortality in coronary artery disease are summarized in Table 1. It must be emphasised that only trials meeting the criteria of adequate design in terms of placebo control, blindness and defined end-points are included. The numerous studies of the symptomatic evaluation of these agents in angina pectoris, cardiac arrhythmias and essential hypertension are excluded. The table is based on an extensive review of the literature (Yusuf et al. 1985) and this should be referred to for the arguments attesting to the validity of the conclusions stated in this paper.

There were sixteen studies with adequate performance criteria involving 16,347 patients, in which beta blockers were given orally, commencing some days after the inscription event. Thirteen of these sixteen prophylactic studies gave negative results, but

---

* 'Atromid' and 'Inderal' are trade marks, the property of Imperial Chemical Industries PLC.

Table 1. Studies of effect of beta blockers on cardiac mortality (based on Yusuf et al. 1985)

Type	Trial number	No. of patients	Outcome
Long-term oral late intervention	16	16,347	13 trials negative 3 trials positive*
Long-term iv + oral early intervention	8	3,582	7 negative 1 positive (?)
Total	24	19,929	Deaths reduced by 20% (p > 0.0001)
Short-term iv + oral early intervention	2	23,000	To be reported in 1985

* Only trials with more than 2,000 patients and over 200 events

three gave positive results in favour of the intervention. An additional eight studies, in which the beta blocker was given parenterally followed by oral administration, showed that only one gave a possible beneficial effect, with seven negative studies. Yet if all the data are pooled so that the results of studies in a total of 19,929 patients are compared, then beta blockade had a highly significant beneficial effect in reducing mortality due to myocardial infarction (p > 0.0001). In general, the risk of death is reduced from about 9.9% to 7.9%, which means that the total number of deaths is reduced by 20%. The pooled data also indicate that sudden death is reduced by 30% (p > 0.00001). Furthermore, the pooled data indicate that long-term treatment with beta blockers reduces the chances of reinfarction by about 25%. There are currently several additional beta blocking studies in progress, the two most important being designed to examine the effect of short-term parenteral/oral beta blockade on long-term survial. These two studies using atenolol ('Tenormin')* and metoprolol ('Lopressor') involved 23,000 patients and the results will become available within the next year.

Studies with hypolipidaemic agents

There are two primary intervention studies and nineteen secondary intervention studies designed to examine the effects of reducing serum cholesterol on morbidity and mortality in coronary artery disease. The agents used for primary intervention were clofibrate in the WHO study, and cholestyramine in the Lipid Research Clinic's Coronary Primary Prevention Trial (LRC-CPPT) and involved a total of 18,000 subjects (Committee of Principal Investigators 1978 & The Lipid Research Clinic's Coronary Primary Prevention Trial 1984). By definition, these were not patients but were selected by measuring serum cholesterol in over half a million non-patient subjects. The nineteen secondary prevention studies have been carried out in a range of patients with sympto-

---

* 'Tenormin' is a trade mark, the property of Imperial Chemical Industries PLC.

Table 2. Hypolipidaemic trials – primary prevention

	Duration (years)	Treatment		Placebo	Cholesterol mg% at entry	Cholesterol Response %
WHO (Clofibrate)	5.3 (treatment)	Events	167	208	249	8.2–9.2
		Deaths	36	34		
	13.2 (Total observation)	Deaths	308	283		
LRCP (cholestyramine)	7	Events	155	187	291.5	8.0
		Deaths	30	38		

matic coronary artery disease and involve a total of 8,000 subjects. The results of the primary prevention study are summarized in Table 2. The clofibrate study lasted 13.2 years and the conclusions from the results are still debated (Green 1984). There was an excess of all-causes deaths in the clofibrate group and no difference on cardiac deaths. There was a 25% reduction in the incidence of non-fatal myocardial infarction. The entry criteria of a cholesterol of 249 mg% was notably lower than that for the cholestyramine study, where the mean entry cholesterol was 291.5 mg%. In the LRC-CPPT study, which lasted seven years, the cardiac mortality was significantly greater in the placebo than in the treated group and this difference was much greater in the subgroup analysis, where there was good compliance with therapy (LRC-CPPT 1984).

The results from the nineteen secondary prevention studies remain controversial, but in a recent pooling analysis presented at a National Institute of Health Consensus Conference on cholesterol and atherosclerosis, it was concluded that reductions of serum cholesterol by a variety of means reduced cardiovascular mortality (Yusuf 1984). One might tentatively conclude that the interventions of beta blockade and lipid lowering conceived 25 years ago have supported the original hypotheses leading to the development of these drugs. The overall effect on morbidity and mortality is not dramatic, but a 15–20% reduction in annual mortality viewed from an epidemiological public health point of view is potentially a very important contribution.

Lessons for the future

1. Trials design

a) Expectations

The fact that it has taken more than 20 years to generate data to justify the conclusions given above suggests that for the future a more effective evaluation process is required. In the early trials of beta blockers relatively small patient groups were studied. The results in 16 of 21 beta blocking trials were negative or equivocal, yet the interventions are now believed to be effective. The first lesson therefore is that in future the expectation of the effect of drug therapy must be more realistic. The early beta blocking trials postulated a 50% reduction in mortality.

When a 20% reduction in mortality was achieved, this was regarded as an unsatisfactory result, whereas in epidemiological terms it is an important effect. When an innovative drug is conceived there are naturally highly optimistic expectations as to its possible clinical value. In a complex multifactorial pathological condition such as atherosclerosis, it is improbable that a single intervention will cause a dramatic reduction in mortality. If significant, but not dramatic, clinical benefit is to be securely demonstrated, then very reliable results are essential.

b) End-points

For a reliable difference to be shown between the treated and control groups there should be a large number of end-points during a trial period. The term "end-points" in the context of intervention studies in atherosclerotic disease means well defined clinical episodes, such as death, reinfarction or stroke. This will improve the chances of showing a difference and improve the power of the study. A common misconception is that the number of patients in a trial determines the power of that trial. The number of patients required is determined by the likelihood of the number of events that are likely to occur, and this determines the reliability of the outcome of the study.

If this principle is applied to the twenty-four trials of beta blockers examining their effects on cardiac morbidity and mortality, twenty-one studies were either negative or equivocal (Table 1). In these twenty-one studies there were less than a total of 150 deaths per trial, and of these twenty-one trials, six reported an unfavourable trend and fifteen a favourable trend. In the three large trials, in which there were more than 150 deaths, all showed a beneficial effect of the intervention at the $p < 0.05$ level. Pooling the twenty-four trials data gives a highly favourable result (Yusuf et al. 1985).

Future studies in cardiovascular disease will have to reach a compromise between those factors favouring a high incidence of events (i.e. age, severity of disease) and the possibility of the intervention being capable of halting or reversing the atherosclerotic process.

c) Considerable biological effect

In regard to future drugs, it will be very desirable that they exert a large predictable biological effect. In the primary prevention lipid lowering studies the original intention was that serum cholesterol should be lowered by between 25–30%. In many of the studies the reduction achieved lay between 6–10% only. Thus, an agent that predictably and consistently reduced serum cholesterol by 30% should have a much greater chance of reducing cardiovascular and morbid events. When the two primary prevention hypolipidaemic trials are compared against the criteria of a large biological effect and an appropriate total incidence of events, it is clear that they have marked shortcomings. In the clofibrate trial, 15,000 volunteer subjects were selected and studied for 13.2 years (Table 2). There were a total of 70 deaths over a 5.3 year treatment period. In the case of the LRC-CPPT cholestyramine study, 3,000 subjects free of symptomatic coronary artery disease were studied for seven years, and there were 30 deaths in the treated group versus 38 in the control group, with a corresponding 155 versus 187 cardiovascular events. Thus, in a total of 20,000 subjects, there was a sub-optimal event incidence. The lesson is that if a very healthy population is studied enormous numbers of subjects are required to generate the likely number of morbid events which, on statistical grounds, should be greater than a total of 650. Furthermore, the entry cholesterol level in the clofibrate study was only 249 mg% and the overall cholesterol reduction was between 8.2 and 9.2%. If there had been a powerful consistent response a much greater reduction in cholesterol would have resulted, and it now seems probable that a beneficial effect would have been detected.

2. Data collection: how much detail?

The considerations summarized above lead to the conclusion that for the future large numbers of patients will need to be studied so that a satisfactory number of end-points occur during the study. To study large numbers over a short period a compromise will be required between the number of patients, the cost and the time involved. In the LRC-CPPT study, it is estimated that the ten year period of evaluation cost $ 150 M, yet the number of end-points was still sub-optimal. In future, a compromise will have to be struck between the degree of patient characterization (480,000 men were screened in the LRC-CPPT study) and applying the intervention to the most suitable patient population sample. There are two potential disadvantages to a policy of large numbers/ minimal data collection.

Firstly, it may not be possible to prove that the treated and control groups are correctly balanced and sufficient data may not be available for sub-group analysis. The concept is that if there is a total event incidence in excess of 650, then this will outweigh any possible influence of small differences between groups, as long as the entry criteria are definite and the end-points unarguable, i.e. death, infarct or stroke.

Sub-group analysis can only give guidance as to what new questions one might wish to address and the disadvantages of retrospective data dredging are now well recognised. The second objection is that side effects due to the intervention may go undetected because of minimal data collection. A possible solution to this could be to ensure that the subject lists any complaints that made him seek medical advice. This should detect major side effects, including any unanticipated for the drug. Clearly, if the study is a risk/ benefit trial, then a different design is required and it is not addressing the question of whether the intervention reduces morbidity and mortality in coronary artery disease. The original purpose of the clofibrate study was to determine whether lowering the cholesterol with clofibrate reduces the prevalence of ischaemic heart disease in hyperlipidaemic subjects. Ironically, it was shown that clofibrate reduced the incidence of ischaemic heart disease by 20%, with a 25% reduction in non-fatal myocardial infarction. Furthermore, the reduction in myocardial infarction was greatest in men with the highest cholesterol and in those who had the greatest reduction in cholesterol in response to clofibrate.

Thus, the original aims of the study were met, but the results were completely overshadowed by the observations of the total number of deaths include mortality rates

from all causes in the clofibrate treated trial group exceeded those in the high cholesterol control group, though the age standardized mortality rates were similar in all
three groups. As the authors comment, "The excessive deaths in the treated group has
diverted attention from the fact that the reduction in the high plasma cholesterol would
reduce the incidence of ischaemic heart disease." (WHO Co-operative Trial 1984).

3. Drug: timing and dose

Examination of the early studies of beta blockers given during the peri-infarction period reveals that the incorrect dose of propranolol was given, probably by the wrong
route, for too short a period of time. Thus, if it is desired to block beta receptors optimally as soon as possible, then the parenteral route must be used, because adequate
plasma levels of beta blocker are not obtained by oral administration (Yusuf 1980).
Simple errors such as these continue to be made in designing intervention studies and
attention to such detail is essential.

Consequences

The possible consequences for the future of novel drug intervention for improving the
morbidity and mortality in atherosclerosis can be viewed from several aspects. These
include the view of the pharmaceutical industry, the medical profession, society,
governments and the media.

The pharmaceutical industry

It is currently estimated that the cost of discovering, developing and marketing a new
chemical entity on a world-wide basis is between £ 30 M and £ 100 M, depending
mainly on the duration of the evaluation in preclinical and clinical toxicity. From the
strategic business point of view, it is legitimate to ask what is the likely financial return,
and when will it occur, if say £ 80 M is invested to develop an innovative drug designed
to reduce cardiovascular morbidity and mortality. The answer must be that it is a very
high risk; that the return will be a long time in appearing, and that the extent of financial return will be limited by patent expiry resulting in generic competition.

a) Time constraints

Innovative drug discovery is a lengthy and time (resource) consuming activity. The
constraints of time begin once the patent is published. At that point the basic toxicology of the preferred compound may not be known, yet the world will be appraised of a
new structure and a claimed biological effect. If the drug is to be given for prolonged
periods to man, then a four year toxicological evaluation must be carried out, and clinical studies of longer than one month duration must await the twelve months taken to
carry out and write up a six month toxicity study in two species. Once the drug is in

Table 3. Clofibrate analogues marketed or in late clinical trials

---

Gemfibrozil
Benzafibrate
Fenofibrate
Tiadenol
Ciprofibrate
Alufibrate
Etofibrate

---

clinical evaluation, it is difficult to see in present circumstances how a beneficial effect on cardiovascular morbidity and mortality could be shown in less than eight years. Professor Mitchell cautioned us earlier that medical directors must emphasize to their respective boards that this is not an area for the faint-hearted who would not be prepared to spend "big money". If it takes ten to twelve years from patent publication to proof of efficacy in this condition, with a patent expiration time of 17–20 years, then the wisdom of spending big money, if there is an intention to see a financial return on it, must be seriously questioned.

b) Benefit to competition

The final WHO report on the clofibrate trial states "Similar comprehensive trials are needed to prove the safety of all new and potent drugs as much as their efficacy". This implies a 13 year clinical evaluation programme. Given the 17–20 year patent life for a novel drug, then a 15 year timetable for discovery and development will give little encouragement to a research-based pharmaceutical company. It will however give encouragement to pharmaceutical companies to adopt a wait, see and act policy. This is well illustrated in the case of the clofibrate analogues. These are listed in Table 3. It is salutary to contrast the sales performance of clofibrate with those of patentable analogues, all discovered to be improvements on clofibrate, but acting in an analogous manner. In 1978 the WHO trial was published and stated "Clofibrate cannot be recommended as a lipid lowering for community-wide prevention of ischaemic heart disease". The result of this pronouncement was two-fold. The market for lipid lowering agents of the clofibrate type was increased by 30% in the seven years since then, to over £ 100 M per annum, and the sales of clofibrate have been completely eclipsed. Yet, clofibrate is the only agent shown to reduce morbidity in ischaemic heart disease. This parodoxical state of affairs indicates that agents not shown to reduce morbidity and mortality in ischaemic heart disease, but shown solely to reduce cholesterol, are to be preferred. The WHO clofibrate trial proved the cholesterol hypothesis and stimulated sales for competitive companies who have not been required to bear the heavy costs of development and proof of efficacy.

c) Future research

Anyone responsible for the strategic investment of many millions of pounds annually in research and development must ponder these observations carefully, in the face of the time constraints, the inappropriately short patent life in relationship to development times, and the competitive advantage to be gained by allowing someone else to do the innovation with the less costly policy of rapid exploitation once the discovery is announced. The policy for continuing to invest in order to discover innovative drugs in atherosclerosis could be made more attractive if the agent had, in addition, an interim beneficial effect. Thus, in the case of the beta blockers, the fact that they are of proven value in angina pectoris, hypertension and cardiac arrhythmias means that an acceptable financial return can be obtained whilst awaiting the results of prolonged studies on morbidity and mortality. New agents that have, for example, just a biological action, such as reducing coagulation abnormalities or decreasing lipids, both of which are postulated to affect the atherosclerotic process, will require prolonged evaluation, with no intermediate return on investment. It is for considerations such as these that ICI Pharmaceuticals Division has currently withdrawn from research in atherosclerosis, despite its pre-eminent position in the field.

The medical profession

The impact of successful drug intervention studies on the medical practice is difficult to assess. Given that every trial represents a compromise between conflicting needs, not surprisingly there are differing interpretations once the results of studies on morbidity and mortality in atherosclerosis are published. Each trial publication triggers a deluge of annotations and review articles. In the beta blocking area, I can detect a ratio of 6–10 review articles per original paper. I have much sympathy for the clinician who wishes to know the state of the art, rather than witness the polemics indulged in by the medical journals. The results of the Norwegian Multi-centre Study on the effect of timolol or morbidity and mortality in survivors of myocardial infarction is an interesting example. This study, which cost several million dollars and necessitated the selection of 3,000 patients out of a population of 11,000, to be studied over two years, resulted in a highly statistically significant reduction in mortality, especially in sudden death. Nevertheless, one reviewer wrote in a medical journal, "If the timolol result carries a one in a thousand chance of a type I error (assuming benefit where none exists) is it not mandatory rather than unethical to repeat the Norwegian trial?" (Mitchell 1981). A year later a different reviewer in the same journal wrote, "It is now clear that beta blockade, used correctly, can prevent many deaths after infarction." (Rose 1982). The busy clinician wishing to apply the results of intervention studies must be confused and frustrated.
Recently, Baber (Baber et al. 1984) carried out a survey of British consultant cardiologists to determine their utilisation of beta blockers following myocardial infarction. They found that 72% of British cardiologists said that they used beta blockers prophylactically, despite the absence of other indications. However, a study of the prescribing habits of general practitioners suggests that there is little increase in the prescribing of beta blockers for ischaemic heart disease. As far as the medical profession in general is concerned, despite studies in over 40,000 patients, there is still no consensus as to which beta blocker should be given to which patient, when it should be started, and for how long it should be continued. It is probable that we will never obtain precise answers to such questions. I would conclude that in general the consequences of the

long-term studies of drug intervention on morbidity and mortality as far as the medical profession is concerned is "mild, positive interest".

Society, governments and the media

Society relies for its information primarily on the media. The media are motivated by the need for news, drama and conflict. Thus, a drug that possibly caused seven deaths amongst 14,000 patients treated for serious ventricular arrhythmias was reported as a near disaster. The fact that the beta blocking study showed a 20–25% reduction in mortality in survivors of infarction is not seen to be newsworthy, though in epidemiological public health terms it is of considerable importance. Similarly, the Medical News headline, "Clofibrate trial proves ill-effects" hardly conveys the impression that clofibrate caused a 25% reduction in re-infarction rate in symptomless hyperlipidaemic subjects.
The issues of relative risk and modest, but important, scientific advances are too complex and arid to capture the attention of the media industry, whose shock/horror "hype" approach to health issues is far removed from the need for balanced education of society. Scientific progress comprises mainly small but important advances in a beneficial direction. The fact that risk assessment can only ever be subjective relating each individual's evaluation of utility and benefit is unappreciated by the media writers. They have no doubt apparently that their value systems relating risk to benefit represent those of society as a whole. Until the media come to terms with these complex un-newsworthy issues, society will continue to be confused and misinformed in the health care area.
The attitude of politicians and governments to proof of therapeutic benefit by drug intervention is not certain or documented. Economic factors now predominate in governmental thinking about therapy. Giving drugs to reduce the morbidity and mortality associated with atherosclerosis will cost more money in an area of already escalating costs. Unless these costs are contained, it is estimated that in the USA 17% of the gross national product may be spent on health care in 1992. Clearly, no politician could admit that advances in therapy are unwelcome, but that is different from giving commitment to ensure that optimal benefit is obtained by applying the results of studies proving efficacy. I suggest that the results of the 25 years' endeavour to evaluate the effects of beta blockers and of hypolipidaemic agents on morbidity and mortality in atherosclerosis are only of the most modest interest to the media and politicians, but are important to society.

Conclusion

The important lessons to be learned from the long-term studies of these agents are:
1. The need to improve drug evaluation techniques as described.
2. The role of elevated cholesterol in atherosclerosis is proven, vindicating the original purpose of Thorp's work (Thorp 1963).
3. The role of inappropriate sympatho-adrenal activity in ischaemic heart disease is established, thus after 25 years supporting the original hypothesis of Black (Black 1967).

4. Future innovative drug research to ameliorate the widespread effects of atherosclerosis will be lengthy, very costly, with little guarantee of an acceptable financial return.
5. The current achievements have had minimal impact on society, the media and
   government.

Acknowledgements

I would like to acknowledge the advice and comment from Dr. Richard Peto in the
preparation of this paper.

References

1. Baber NS, Julian DG, Lewis JA, Rose G (1984) Beta blockers after myocardial infarction:
   have trials changed practice? Br Med J 289:1431–1432
2. Black JW (1967) The predictive value of animal tests in relation to drugs affecting the cardiovascular system in man. In: Drug Responses in Man, J & A Churchill Ltd, London, p 113
   and pp 121–122
3. Committee of Principal Investigators (1978) A co-operative trial in the prevention of
   ischaemic heart disease using clofibrate. Br Heart J 40:1069–1118
4. Fitzgerald JD (1972) The role of beta-adrenergic blockade in acute myocardial ischaemia. In:
   Oliver MF, Julian DG, Donald KW (eds) Effect of Acute Ischaemia in Myocardial Function.
   Churchill Livingstone, Edinburgh & London, pp 321–353
5. Green KG (1984) Interpretation of Clofibrate Trial. Lancet II:1095–1096
6. The Lipid Research Clinic's Coronary Primary Prevention Trial Results (1984) II. The Relationship of Reduction in Incidence of Coronary Heart Disease to Cholesterol Lowering.
   JAMA 251:365–374
7. Mitchell JRA (1981) Timolol after myocardial infarction: an answer or a new set of questions?
   Br Med J 282:1565–1570
8. The Norwegian Multi-centre Study Group (1981) Timolol-induced Reduction in Mortality and
   Reinfarction in Patients Surviving Acute Myocardial Infarction. Engl J Med 304:801–807
9. Rose G (1982) Should every survivor of a heart attack be given a beta-blocker? Part III. Some
   conclusions. Br Med J 285:39–40
10. WHO Co-operative Trial on Primary Prevention of Ischaemic Heart Disease with Clofibrate
    to Lower Serum Cholesterol (1984) Final Mortality Follow-up. Report of the Committee on
    Principal Investigators. Lancet II:600–604
11. Yusuf S (1980) Beta-adrenergic blockade in acute myocardial infarction. D Phil Thesis, Ox-
    ford University
12. Yusuf S (1984) Personal communication to NIH Consensus Conference
13. Yusuf S, Peto R, Lewis J, Collins R, Sleight P (1985) Beta blockade during and after myo-
    cardial infarction: an overview of the randomised trials. Prog Cardiovasc Dis (in press)

Author's address:
J. D. Fitzgerald, M.D.
Imperial Chemical Industries PLC
Pharmaceuticals Division
Alderley Park
Macclesfield
Cheshire, SK10 4TF, Great Britain

Discussion

FITZGERALD

A listener who had himself taken part in a long-term intervention study stated that more attention needs to be given to the consequences of stopping such trials. Are patients who have been treated for many years with aspirin or beta blockers at excess risk when they have their medication discontinued? A plea was made for including a randomized stopping procedure and longer periods of follow-up in intervention trials.

Rauwolfia derivatives and breast cancer: how do we know when we have the answers?

C. R. B. Joyce

Introduction

The problem of combining results from different centres or different experiments is faced by biometricians of the pharmaceutical industry and their clinical colleagues every day. Pressures on limited resources, even in diseases with high incidence or morbidity, have long made the multicentre trial an unwelcome methodological fixture. A great deal more could still be said about the strengths and weaknesses of the techniques used to make the inferences from n patients spread among m centres as strong as – or stronger than – those from nm patients treated in a single centre. A problem that, although it has some properties in common with those of the multicentre trial, seems to have received rather less attention or even to have been almost entirely neglected by some of those whom it most concerns is the combination of information from studies that are spread out not only in space but also in time.

This situation is true of attempts to answer any scientific question that has more than trivial implications; but the intention of this paper is to illustrate the nature of the problem in regard to adverse reactions. That, unfortunately, takes more and more of the time of workers in the drug industry at the expense of truly creative work. As is well known, the causal attribution of adverse events that are infrequent, long delayed in onset, or occur on a high base-line of a similar disease can very seldom be achieved by prospective study, which (virtually by definition) takes too long and/or too many patients and is also likely to be unethical (the deliberate provocation of serious toxicity in man is not a permissible activity for civilised people). But more and more often, every lesion in rats treated for two years with doses many times in excess of those considered for therapeutic use is considered to demonstrate a long-term risk to humans receiving any dose at all. Answers to questions about the association of drug and delayed or severe effects in human beings are demanded by authorities as well as managers of the industry. This demand has been partially met by the development of epidemiological methods, of which the case-control study is the best-known and most frequently used.

A paper from the Boston Collaborative Drug Surveillance Program (BCDSP 1974) originally generated the hypothesis of an association between the ingestion of rauwolfia alkaloids and the subsequent development of breast cancer. The problem posed by the title of this paper will be illustrated with a commentary on the series of studies to which this hypothesis gave rise.

Background

The BCDSP makes use of a network of hospitals, mainly in North America, to record drug use and clinical responses of in-patients. Patients are also asked to recall their use of therapeutic agents during the previous six months.

The resulting diagnostic and treatment data bases are used to identify associations between specific diseases and recorded use of any drug. Given the very large size of the data base and the number of associations examined, many statistically significant correlations will appear by chance, even if they have no basis in clinical reality. Such a "completely unexpected" correlation between breast cancer in women and use of "reserpine" (in fact, rauwolfia alkaloids) was identified in this way by the BCDSP in 1974. Many authors (including those of the first paper) have referred to an association between breast cancer and "reserpine" rather than "rauwolfia alkaloids", of which reserpine is only one – although, in fact, the most widely used. It is not only poor science to describe the subject of study incorrectly, but it is also invalid to apply data, relating to one substance, uncritically to another. Specifically, it cannot be assumed without appropriate testing that all structural analogues dervied from rauwolfia would be carcinogenic, still less that they would be equipotent as carcinogens. The fact that only some of the observations are relevant to reserpine itself therefore weakens the case against it, but there are many other difficulties.

From the observation that women with diagnosed breast cancer reported previous medication with rauwolfia alkaloids more often than women in a control group, the hypothesis was proposed that women medicated with "reserpine" (sic) had an increased risk of developing breast cancer. This was tested against two other contemporary hospitalised groups of patients, one surgical, the other medical. Like the breast cancer cases, these were already part of the data base from which the hypothesis had been generated and so could not be used to provide a fully independent test. However, the hypothesis was apparently supported by two other studies that were published simultaneously (Armstrong et al. 1974, Heinonen et al. 1974).

At least 21 further epidemiological studies of this question are known to have been carried out after the first 3, of which the results of 20 have been published, 18 of them in full (see Table 1). At least 2 papers that failed to confirm the initial hypothesis, one of which was of major importance, were initially refused publication, the journal editors stating, respectively, that "enough has been published on this subject by now" and that there was no need to publish a full paper on negative results. The latter was eventually published elsewhere; so far as is known, the former has never been published at all. All but 5 have used retrospective case-control methodology. (An abstract by Farber and Detels (1977) is based on a doctoral thesis by Farber in which a prospective trial, a cohort study and a case-control study were carried out on the same population.)

Major problems of retrospective case-control studies

The possibilities for testing such hypotheses and quantifying their consequences are limited. The *attributable risk ratio,* which compares the *incidence* of breast cancer in women who have received rauwolfia alkaloids with that in otherwise similar women not so exposed, and so enables the excess "attributable" to the drug to be calculated, requires either a prospective study or complete knowledge of relevant medication and disease in a closed population of adequate size. Breast cancer is infrequent (the average age-corrected annual incidence in women at risk is 0.1%) and the alleged consequence may take years to develop. The more practical retrospective case-control method yields a *relative risk ratio,* which compares the *frequency* with which cases of breast cancer

90

Table 1. Summary of reported risk ratios

No.	First author	(Ref.)	Country	Type of study	Relative risk ratio (95% confidence limits)*	Authors' interpretation
1	BCDSP	(4)	USA (Massachusetts)	Case-Control	(Generated hypothesis of association: not independently tested)	
2	Armstrong	(2)	UK	Case-Control	2.0 (0.74–5.5)	+ Statistically significant association
3	Heinonen	(12)	SF	Case-Control	2.0 (1.2 –3.4)	+ Positive association
4	Mack	(26)	USA (California)	Case-Control	1.2 (0.7 –2.2)	– Do not support the hypothesis
5	O'Fallon	(32)	USA (Minnesota)	Case-Control	0.99 (NA–1.55)	– Association unlikely
6	Miller +	(29)	USA (Tennessee)	Case-Control	0.74	– Risk not significantly different from 1.0
7	Laska	(24)	USA (New York)	Case-Control	1.1	– No significant increased relative risk
8	Simpson +	(35)	NZ	Cohort	–	? Inconclusive
9	Lilienfeld	(25)	USA (Maryland)	Case-Control	Hospital Controls: 1.6 (0.85–2.9) Neighbourhood Controls: 0.88 (0.44–1.7)	– Reserpine not risk factor for breast cancer
11	Armstrong	(1)	UK	Case-Control	2.1 (0.94–4.9)	+ Positive association
12	Aromaa	(3)	SF	Case-Control	1.0 (0.52–1.9)	– Unlikely that reserpine increases risk
13	Kewitz	(20)	D	Case-Control	0.6 (0.4 –1.1)	– Does not support the hypothesis
14	Christopher	(5)	UK	Case-Control	0.94	– Does not support the hypothesis
15	Jus + +	(19)	CDN	Cohort	1.3	– No significant exposure
16	Kodlin	(21)	USA (California)	Case-Control	1.1	– Fails to support suspicions of causality
17	Williams	(39)	USA (Maryland)	Case-Control	2.0	+ Significant low level association
18	Watanuki	(38)	J	Case-Control	–	? Inconclusive
19	Moriwaki	(30)	J	Case-Control	–	? Inconclusive
20	Takatani +	(36)	J	Case-Control	–	– No statistically significant association
21	Labarthe	(23)	USA (Minnesota)	Cohort	1.02 (0.51–1.82)	– No evidence of any association
22	Curb	(6)	USA	Cohort	1.28 (0.58–2.80)	– No evidence of association
23	Friedman	(10)	USA (California)	Cohort	0.9 (0.4 –2.1)	– Hypothesis could not be confirmed
24	Shapiro	(34)	USA (Massachusetts)	Case-Control	0.7 (0.5 –1.0)	– Original association probably due to chance
25	Farber +	(8)	USA (California)	Prosp., cohort, c-c		– None of the 3 studies gave support

   * Except 2 (90%) and 5 (99%)
  + Abstract only
+ + Unpublished

and appropriate controls were previously exposed to rauwolfia alkaloids. The difference in the information provided by the two methods and the calculations they permit of the types of risk cannot be over-emphasized. Only the *prospective* (or cohort) experiment, as a rule, allows an answer to the question of chief interest: *Has a patient receiving rauwolfia alkaloids an increased risk of developing breast cancer?* The retrospective (case-control) analysis answers the suggestive but tangential question: *Is a woman with breast cancer more likely to have been previously treated with rauwolfia alkaloids?* The great majority (17/23, if that by Farber and Detels (1977) is ignored) of studies of the problem have been attempts to answer the second question.

Comments on the series of studies

The major features of all 24 studies are summarized in Tables 1–6. Three were inconclusive, but the authors of all but 4 of the remainder considered that their results

Table 2. Relevant preparations specifically included in study

---

Case-control studies

No. 1. Reserpine-containing drugs: unbranded reserpine, Serpasil, Ser-Ap-Es, Diupres, Rauzide, Hydropres

2. Rauwolfia derivatives: reserpine, standardized rauwolfia alkaloids, methoserpidine, deserpidine

3. Reserpine, rauwolfia alkaloids, or any drug containing reserpine, rescinnamine, or rauwolfia alkaloids

4. Rauwolfia preparations, rauwolfia serpentina, reserpine

5. Rauwolfia agents: whole-root rauwolfia and reserpine

6. Rauwolfia alkaloids

7. All medications containing rauwolfia

9. Rauwolfia preparations

11. Rauwolfia derivatives

12. Rauwolfia derivatives

13. Rauwolfia-containing preparations, mostly in fixed combination

14. Rauwolfia derivatives

16. Preparations containing reserpine

17. Nominally reserpine

18. Several kinds of reserpine

19. Rauwolfia serpentina

20. Rauwolfia derivatives

24. Rauwolfia Alkaloids

Cohort studies

No. 8. Rauwolfia drugs

15. Reserpine

21. Any reserpine-related agents

22. Reserpine

23. Rauwolfia derivatives, including combinations

N.B. All Reference nos. are to Table 1, Col. 1.

Table 3. Selected inclusion and exclusion characteristics of cases and controls

Case-control studies

No. 1. *Cases*
First diagnosis, from 25,000 hospitalized patients in Boston area, 1972; 159 new cases; 9 with inadequate drug history excluded $n=150$
Controls, surgical
6,500 candidates; 309 with other cancers, 180 with inadequate drug history excluded; 10% sample for 4:1 match by decade of age, hospital $n=600$
Controls, medical
5,200 candidates, 1,686 with cardiovascular diseases or other cancer and 171 with inadequate drug history excluded; c. 15% sample for 4:1 match $n=600$

2. *Cases*
First diagnosis, 750 newly registered cases, 1971–1973; 32 with inadequate history excluded $n=708$
Controls, all other cancers
Initially sampled to provide 3:1 match by 5-year age range, year of registration; matched subjects not newly diagnosed or with inadequate history excluded $n=1,430$
Controls, selected other cancers
Subset of above after exclusion of subjects with cancers of pancreas, skin, corpus uteri, kidney, nervous system $n=963$

3. *Cases*
First diagnosis, mastectomy for breast cancer in a Helsinki hospital, 1960–1972; those with any other cancer or inadequate history in case or paired control excluded $n=438$
Controls, surgical
Subjects with elective surgery and not cancer; those with surgery for gall bladder, thyroid or kidney disease, cardiac or vascular surgery or sympathectomy or inadequate history excluded; matched by 5-year age interval and year of surgery, 1:1 $n=438$

4. *Cases*
120 notifications to health facility or surveillance agency of breast cancer, 1971–1975; 2 with breast metastases, 7 lacking records excluded; in most analyses those with prior breast cancer and other cancers also excluded $n=99$
Controls, community residents
Roster searched for age and community-entry matches within 6 months, subjects without charts or with benign breast disease excluded $n=444\ or\ 396$

5. *Cases*
First diagnosis, 453 breast cancers ($>1/3$ hypertensive) from defined population, diagnosed 1955–1973, 3 with inadequate history excluded $n=450$
Controls, gall bladder disease (1/2 hypertensive)
Stratified sample from 2,000 subjects, diagnosed 1955–1970 to match age distribution of cases; no exclusions $n=475$

6. *Cases*
First diagnosis $n=247$
Controls, colonic cancer $n=108$

7. *Cases*
55 cases with breast cancer diagnosed while resident in institution, 1965–1974, on average 18 years before diagnosis; no exclusions $n=55$
Controls
55 controls matched on age, psychiatric diagnosis, admission date, (sometimes) race and religion; all resident in hospital April 1, 1969; no exclusions $n=55$

9. *Cases*
273 new histologically diagnosed patients without previous primary breast malignancy in Breast Tumor Collaborative Study, 1973–January 1974; 38 without interview, 39 with inadequate history in case or matched control excluded; 32 not matched with hospital control; 57 not matched with neighbourhood control
$n = 164$
(matched to hospital control)
$n = 139$
(matched to neighbourhood control)

Controls, hospital
242 patients matched by sex, within 5 years of age; residence, race, hospital service, date of admission; free of prior breast cancer; 30 with no interview, 48 with inadequate history excluded
$n = 164$

Controls, neighbourhood
201 subjects with similar demographic matching; 35 without interviews and 27 with inadequate history excluded
$n = 139$

11. *Cases*
58 patients with death certificates in special analysis samples (10% of 1972, 25% of 1973), with all diagnoses coded, including breast cancer and hypertension; 11 with inadequate history excluded
$n = 47 (33, 35)$

Controls, other cancers
105 patients with other cancers and hypertension found when seeking match for year of death, 5-year age interval at death; 14 with inadequate history excluded
$n = 91 (76)$

Controls, no cancer
254 patients identified as above; 71 with inadequate history excluded
$n = 183 (97)$

12. *Cases*
126 patients record-linked in Finnish Cancer Registry and Social Insurance programme, breast cancer reported in 1973, antihypertensive medications reimbursed by 1972; 7 pairs where case or control lacked adequate history excluded
$n = 109$

Controls, other hypertensives
Selected from among 3 provisional controls per case after matching by geographic area, age (one year), and duration of hypertension
$n = 109$

13. *Cases*
526 women admitted to any of 20 hospitals for breast biopsy, having no other cancer; 336 without breast cancer on biopsy and 9 over 80 years old
$n = 181$

Controls, benign breast disease
Remainder of cancer-free biopsy series; 29 under 30 years old excluded
$n = 307$

Controls, other surgery
Other surgical patients, excluding those with gall bladder disease or any cancer
$n = 101$

14. *Cases*
All discharge diagnoses of breast cancer 1969–1974: Aberdeen, *646* matched sets with 2 controls each; Dundee, *233* matched sets with 2 controls each; Hammersmith, *116* matched sets; total
$n = 996$

Controls, other cancer
Combined Aberdeen and Dundee controls age-matched; total
$n = 879$

Controls, cardiac rematch
Combined controls after replacement of all cardiac diagnoses (n = 102); total
$n = 996$

16. *Cases*
(a) 789 breast cancers diagnosed 1964–1973 reported to Tumour Registry or indexed in hospital records 1974–1975; 108/143 had evidence confirmed of hypertension before cancer (BP > 160/> 90)
$n = 108$

(b) 433 women who had »Multiphasic Health Check-up (MHC)« at least once between 1964–1973
Controls
From 250,000 hospital records, 20 potential controls per case selected by computer; matched for race, year of MHC and age ± 1 year at MHC; 3 controls/case   *n = 324*
Covariates
Age at diagnosis of hypertension, interval to diagnosis of breast cancer, obesity, parity, education

17. *Cases*
New breast cancer cases in national screening programme matched for biopsied women with negative histology, within five years of age, race, screening centre, if possible to within six months of entry to screening project   *n = 543*
Controls
(a) Negative screen   *n = 1,422*
(b) Positive screen but negative biopsy   *n = 481*

18. *Cases*
Breast cancer in 55 institutions, April–December 1975   *n = 1,707*
Controls
Mastopathy, fibroadenoma, etc.   *n = 4,323*

19. *Cases*
From 500 breast cancers surgically treated in one hospital October 1966–December 1976   *n = 402*
Controls
76 gynaecomastia, 470 cervical cancer, 300 female gastric cancer, 6 male breast cancer   *n = 852*

20. *Cases*
4 hospitals (September 1975–November 1977)   *n = 1,000*
Controls
Other diseases   *n = c. 2,500*

24. *Cases*
All new (< 6 m.) breast cancer diagnoses w.o. other primary or previous cancer   *n = 1,881*
Controls
Benign conditions not related to antihypertensive drug use, no history of cancer   *n = 1,523*

Cohort studies
No. 8. All patients attending hypertension clinic earlier than 1966, followed ≧ 4 years, developing malignancy ≧ 4 years from first attendance or starting treatment   *treated n = 359*
          untreated n = 103

15. Hospitalized mental patients 1954–1969; follow-up until 1975   *treated n = 724*
          untreated n = 7,287

21. *Cases*
Review of Rochester Epidemiology Project Record Linkage System first diagnosed 1950–1969. ≧ 6 m. follow-up; definite reserpine exposure ≧ 1 yr.   *n = 250*
Controls
Expected incidence from (1) Olmsted County, (2) Connecticut Tumour Registry

22. *Cases*
HDFP »stepped-care« group receiving reserpine, 5 yr. follow-up   *n = 1,036*
Controls
HDFP »stepped-care« group never receiving reserpine, 5 yr. follow-up   *n = 1,493*

Table 3. Continued

---

23. *Cases*
    Subscribers to Kaiser-Permanente Medical Care Programme known receiving rauwolfia
    between 1969–1973 $n = 2,365$
    Controls
    Entire drug-user cohort
    Also 5 per case, age decade matched, to test subsidiary hypotheses, using rauwolfia w.o.
    breast cancer

---

did not support the original hypothesis. Differences in the major features of the populations examined, the sample sizes and methods of ascertaining and recording observations may have been in part responsible for these disparities, but they can hardly have been solely responsible for depriving the hypothesis of so much support.

The estimate of the relative risk contained in the first report (BCDSP 1974) was the highest recorded. More recently, however, one of the original members of the BCDSP, using the same methods and, by this time, a much larger available population of patient records, was unable to confirm the original BCDSP hypothesis (Shapiro et al. 1984). The authors of the later report considered that the original findings were due to chance effects in a sample of inadequate size.

The second group of investigators, on first analysis of the data, could not find a statistically significant excess use of rauwolfia alkaloids in women with diagnosed breast cancer (Armstrong et al. 1974). The data were re-analyzed after excluding all patients who had other cancers alleged, but not recessarily reported, by the BCDSP to be associated with "reserpine". Statistical significance was then attained. However, the same group of investigators was subsequently (Armstrong et al. 1976) unable to confirm the alleged association of rauwolfia alkaloids with cancers other than of the breast. They thus invalidated the exclusions in their original study and, consequently, its conclusions (compare Armstrong et al. 1974 and Armstrong et al. 1976).

The authors of the third paper (Heinonen et al. 1974) included members of the BCDSP. It is not clear that safeguards against observer bias were as rigorous as those used by the BCDSP (1974); and inconsistencies in the data, particularly in regard to relationships with time, were difficult to interpret.

Neither the case-control nor the cohort design is able to allocate patients randomly to the treatments of interest. In consequence, the machinery of chance cannot be relied upon to take its usual automatic care of such factors, in the problem under review, as age, parity, dose and duration of treatment, etc., that may otherwise be distributed unequally between the groups and confuse the interpretation of important differences between them. Such control must be achieved in other ways. Even when, as is rarely possible, the cases are drawn from a closed group (such as a retirement community), so that a control (non-breast cancer) sample can be taken from the identical population, it will generally be necessary to *match* each case on known "risk factors", including those mentioned above, with at least one control. Up to 4 or even more controls are often matched to each case, in order to increase the security of such matching, and perhaps to allow for the role of other potential but undetermined risk factors. The published list of these continues to increase; it already includes, for breast cancer, factors as diverse

Table 4. Ascertainment of medication with rauwolfia alkaloids

Case-control studies

No. 1. In-hospital interview on use of medication during 3 months before admission; if response positive for treatment of high blood pressure, identity, frequency and duration of use of antihypertensive medications sought

2. (1) GP admission form; (2) admission medical history; (3) project-initiated; (4) GP practice notes searched in sequence until exhausted or adequate data obtained. If rauwolfia derivatives identified, GP notes sought for dose and duration

3. Medical record sources linked to current hospitalization; prior use information limited to referral letters, outpatient notes, current and previous admission histories, in-patient drug records, anaesthetic records and consultants' notes

4. Outpatient clinic records, including general medical history recorded at entry to community, possibly including pre-entry drug use

5. Outpatient and inpatient medical records

6. No information

7. Inpatient medical records

9. Interview response to enquiry whether ever hypertensive; if yes, when and by whom treated; letters to physicians named plus search of clinic records when participating hospital involved; interview response linked to hospital admission for cases and hospital controls, not neighbourhood controls; only 2/3 of interviews completed in hospital

11. GP records

12. Social Insurance records of reimbursement for medications purchased during 1972, giving name, amount purchased and dosage for all purchases; physicians contacted to determine duration of hypertension

13. If in-hospital response positive for »regular use for at least three months«, dosage, duration of treatment and between-treatment intervals sought. If history positive for hypertension, questionnaire sent to physician for similar data on antihypertensive and other cardiovascular drugs

14. Hospital records at admission plus request for supplemental information (at Hammersmith, no hospital history for controls)

16. Review of case records of all confirmed hypertensives

17. Postal patient questionnaires on medication for diabetes, hypertension, ankle oedema and thyroid disease – control questions on medication for birth control or menopause
Each physician named by patient received questionnaire to confirm diagnosis of hypertension or edema, and therapy. Response rate: 88% patients, 73% physicians

18. Questionnaire to institutions: »drugs uncertain in nearly half of 204 cases«

19. Clinical records

20. Questionnaire to doctors consulted by patients

24. As for study 1; *lifetime* drug history

Cohort studies

No. 8. No information

10. »Detailed drug history«

15. Hospital files

21. Detailed review of Rochester Record Linkage System data

22. Extensive search of hospital and clinic records of patients in HDFP programme

23. Computer-stored prescription records from San Francisco Kaiser-Permanente pharmacy

Table 5. Criteria for identification of patient as user of rauwolfia alkaloids

---

Case-control studies

No. 1. Any positive history = user (current)
Further analysis by duration of use (1, 1–3, 4–5, 5+ years)

2. Any positive history = user (current)

3. Any positive history = user (ever)

4. Any positive history = user (ever)
Separate analysis for users ≧ 5 years before diagnosis

5. Positive history ≧ 6 months before diagnosis = user (ever)
Further analyses by interval from first use to diagnosis (1, 2, 3, . . ., 8, 9, 10+ years)

6. No information

7. Any positive history = user (ever)
Further analyses by years of use of ≧ 25 mg, relative to year of diagnosis; cumulative years; mean number of days and mean dosage

9. Any positive history = user (ever)
Further analyses by average dose per user and average duration of use per user

11. Any positive history = user (ever)
Further analyses by use before cancer diagnosis, before and after, after only, any period ≧ 3 months before diagnosis, any period ≧ 5 years before diagnosis

12. Any positive history = user (recent)
Additional analysis as »main« antihypertensive agent (use – days as other agents)

13. Any positive history = user (ever)
Further analyses by duration of use ≦ 1 year, proximity of use to date of diagnosis (within same year), use for ≧ 1 years up to the time of diagnosis

14. Any positive history = user (ever)
Further analyses by use at time of diagnosis of cancer, ≧ 1 year, 1 year from diagnosis; Aberdeen also grouped at more than 6 months before diagnosis

16. Any usage, use ≧ 1 year and within last three months, use > five years

17. Use ≧ 1 year and ≧ 5 years

18. ?

19. ?

20. ?

24. Apparently similar to study 1

Cohort studies

No. 8. Use ≧ 4 years

10. Average follow-up from first use = 11 years

15. No information

21. »Any«, and 1 yr »definite use according to detailed criteria«

22. Use prescribed by programme; 1 yr. compliance 80% patients taking 80% prescribed medication

23. Received drug according to computerized pharmacy data-base

---

as hair dyes and tonsillectomy. The number of cases studied in the present series of reports varies from 33 to 1,881 and of controls from 55 to 7,287. The ratio of cases to controls varies from approximately 0.3 : 1 to 10 : 1.

As important as the definition of patient characteristics necessary for inclusion in the case and control groups is that of other factors that will imply exclusion. Thus it is clear

98

that no patients with breast cancer should enter the control group; but it is by no means as clear that patients with current diseases – notably those involving hypertension – that could be treated with the drug under suspicion should be excluded.

An inevitable but important further source of many difficulties, as far as case-control studies in particular are concerned, is the fact that, because the collection of the relevant medical information will already have been completed in the course of normal medical practice before the survey is carried out, its quality and comprehensiveness will vary from observer to observer as well as over time, etc. This will be especially true of information about the drugs to which the patient has been exposed, a matter of crucial relevance, and even more so when the patient herself is the sole source of information. In the present series of studies, information on use of rauwolfia and its derivatives was derived from hospital records, the physician's record or patient's recall, methods of respectively increasing fallibility. In addition to this great variability in the number of patients and controls, the definition of diagnosis, duration of exposure to treatment, etc., varied greatly from study to study (Tables 2–6). (The method of summary is that adopted by Labarthe (1979) for the 11 studies available to him at that time.) There was a slight tendency for the *relative* risk ratio to decline over successive studies (Fig. 1). This may have been due in part to increasing precision in the methodology as the deficiencies of earlier publications are identified and reduced. Such variations may also be due to differences in the exact hypothesis under test but must obviously limit direct comparability between different studies.

Some studies also reported elevated relative risk ratios for development of breast cancer in association with exposure to other anti-hypertensive agents as well as with totally unrelated drugs: e.g., phenobarbital (Mack et al. 1975, O'Fallon et al. 1975, Aromaa et al. 1976). Such relationships have even less biological foundation than can be advanced for rauwolfia and therefore increase doubt about the clinical significance of these findings, and the relevance of the methods in general.

Previous reviews

There have been four major independent reviews of the epidemiological evidence (Henderson 1977, Department of Health, Education, and Welfare, (DHEW) 1978, Labarthe 1979, International Agency for Research on Cancer (IARC) 1980). The first 3 appeared between 1977 and 1979, and covered less than half the publications available in 1984. Two were published by individual expert epidemiologists, Henderson and Labarthe, neither of whom considered that the evidence for a causal relationship was sufficient to convince (Henderson 1977, Labarthe 1979). The DHEW Ad Hoc Committee, of which Henderson was Chairman, was – perhaps not surprisingly – unable to agree upon a unanimous report for publication, but considered that a causal relationship was unlikely and the increased risk small, even if real.

The IARC review (1980) of 13 case-control and 2 cohort studies considered the association unlikely, but was unable to exclude the possibility of a slightly increased risk, owing to sampling variation and other methodological difficulties. In fact, the evidence accumulated since the publication of these reviews has not provided additional support either for the original major or subsequent minor hypotheses, which may now perhaps be regarded as decisively lacking support. Particularly relevant are the three recent

Table 6. Some major criticisms of case-control papers

No. 1. *Case selection:* Population base not known; sample too small.
Control, selection and matching: controls from lower socio-economic groups than cases; differential exclusion rates of cases and controls treated with anti-hypertensives unknown; surgical and medical reanalyses indicated wide differences between control groups; »reserpine« users under-represented; population base not known.
Drug and other records: parameters of exposure unclear; combinations included in analysis; patient recall unreliable; drug use only current or very recent.
Confounding, analysis and inference: multiple comparisons; latency short for carcinogenesis; no information on obesity available; testing hypothesis on initial body of data illegitimate.

2. *Case selection:* inclusion of early cases may dilute effect.
Control selection and matching: controls had worse prognosis; exclusions give lower socio-economic class, therefore less medical care than controls; exclusions subsequently demonstrated unjustified; control group all had cancer.
Drug and other records: heterogeneous sources; parameters of exposure unclear; differences in sources for cases and controls; drug use very recent.
Confounding, analysis and inference: method of analysis unpublished; some necessary data and analyses not presented; use of Boston »results« to alter data improper in a confirmatory study.

3. *Case selection:* population base not known.
Control selection and matching: gall bladder disease exclusions invalid; population base not known; major surgery cases nonrepresentative.
Drug and other records: parameters of exposure unclear; records of low quality; checking method inadequate.
Confounding, analysis and inference: methods standardisation with Boston study unwise; reanalysis for hypertension reverses risk ratio.

4. *Case selection:* large number of exclusions.
Control selection and matching: large number of exclusions.
Drug and other records: intermittent »other« drug records unreliable; »other antihypertensive« drug users possibly also reserpine users.
Confounding, analysis and inference: abstracting neither blind nor repeated; low power.

studies using the more powerful cohort methodology (Labarthe and O'Fallon 1980, Curb et al. 1982, Friedman 1983), two of which established ratios not significantly different from unity (Labarthe and O'Fallon 1980, Curb et al. 1982). These have also excluded the alternative possibility, suggested by Williams et al. (1978) of increased incidence associated with long-term use (> 5 years). The contrary hypothesis, of a higher association with recent use, had been put forward by the DHEW Ad Hoc Committee (1978). This was later specifically examined, and excluded, by Friedman (1983); so the evidence concerning duration of use appears to have been rather thoroughly disposed of.

An important additional report of simultaneous prospective, cohort and case-control studies on samples from the same population (Farber and Detels 1977) has unfortunately only ever been reported in abstract. Farber's Ph.D. thesis, on which this communication was based, makes it clear, however, that no increased risk was visible in any of the 3 studies.

Table 6. Continued

____

5. *Case selection:* inclusion of early cases may dilute association.
   Control selection and matching: single diagnostic group as controls did not represent population.
7. *Case selection:* population base not known.
   Control selection and matching: psychiatric patients unsuitable controls if prolactin hypothesis correct; population base not known.
   Drug and other records: drug usage much lower than expected in psychiatric patients.
   Confounding, analysis and inference: small sample; re-analysis showed contrary result; low power.
9. *Drug and other records:* frequent unavailability, physicians non-cooperative; patient self-reporting unreliable.
   Confounding, analysis and inference: low power.
11. *Case selection:* death certification problems.
    Drug and other records: general physician matching essential for differences in practice.
    Confounding, analysis and inference: small numbers; significance achieved only when treatments after breast cancer diagnosis included; comparisons unbalanced with respect to onset of hypertension.
12. *Control selection and matching:* larger number of tentative controls would have matched drug use duration better.
    Confounding, analysis and inference: obesity not controlled.
13. *Drug and other records:* patient self-reporting unreliable.
    Confounding, analysis and inference: hypertension and drug use confounded.
14. *Confounding, analysis and inference:* multicentre problems.
15. *Case selection:* under-reporting to Registry »notorious«; small sample, not randomly selected; significant differences from controls.
    Confounding, analysis and inference: low power.
17. *Case and control selection:* subjects all volunteers.
24. *Drug and other records:* after diagnosis established?

____

Clinical relevance

A causal relationship between the clinical use of rauwolfia alkaloids and the appearance of breast cancer has thus not been demonstrated by the large body of epidemiological evidence now available. Reserpine, especially, is not an obsolete antihypertensive agent. It has been widely used for over 30 years as an effective and well-tolerated antihypertensive. Although prescribing has been considerably (and, as has been shown, inappropriately) reduced since the 1974 reports, it is still used in several European countries, Japan and USA, and has an important place in the therapy of hypertension in third world countries. Its low cost compared with that of other antihypertensive agents is important for patients in countries with limited health resources. Its relatively long duration of action allows it to be given only once a day and this makes patient compliance easier. The clinical evidence for its effectiveness is extensive and will not be reviewed here (Moser 1977, Veterans Administration Cooperative Study

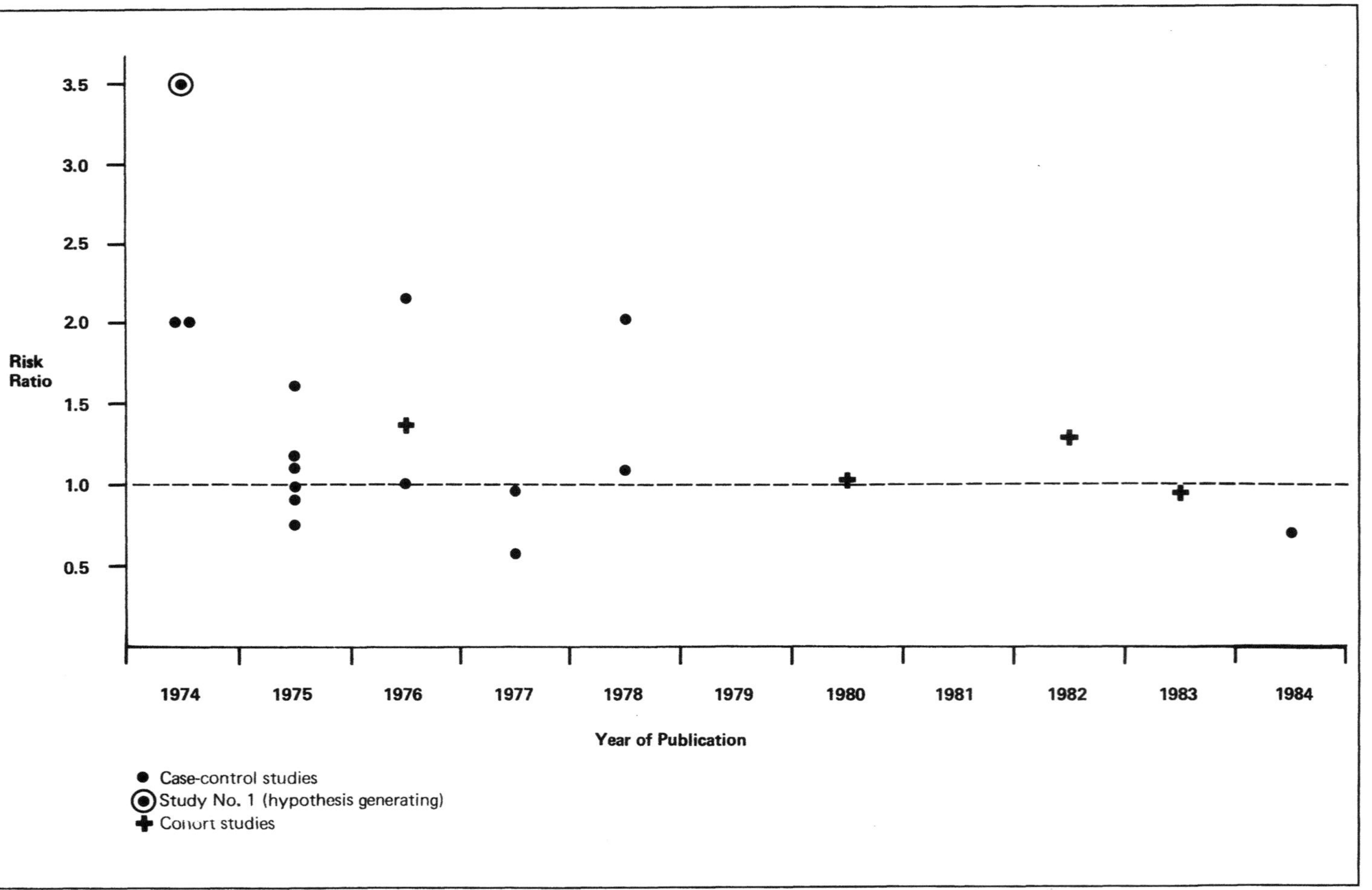

Fig. 1. Main risk estimate and year of publication.

Group 1977, Hypertension Detection and Follow-up Program Cooperative Group 1979, Management Committee of the Australian Trial in Mild Hypertension 1979).

Regulatory events

Although the series of rauwolfia-breast cancer studies did not represent the first application of epidemiological methods to the examination of an alleged drug-adverse event association, it was unusual and important in at least two ways. First, the hypothesis was generated in the course of routine checking of all drugs against all diagnoses in the BCDSP data-banks; second, the series was of an almost unprecedented length that was unnecessary and therefore uneconomical. Even had each study been regarded as contributing only one bit (i.e., binary digit) of information, the likelihood of a set of 20 studies (the initial hypothesis-generating study and the 3 inconclusive being omitted) giving rise to 16 negative and only 4 positive findings by chance, without considering that the association was in fact alleged to be positive, is less than 0.1%. The conventional 5% level of significance was actually obtained at the 13th study, if all are taken in sequential order of publication. The probability did not fall below this level when the single further positive finding was subsequently reported (Williams et al. 1978).
Yet some regulatory authorities came to the wrong conclusion. The FDA reaction, if not typical, was for the usual and obvious reasons the most important. Soon after the publication in September 1974 of the first three papers, the FDA announced, in its Drug Bulletin for that month, that "after review of all the evidence" it would "promptly announce its decision regarding the continued marketing status and labeling".
Many hearings and meetings followed. Following the last public hearings on June 22 and November 19, 1979, and February 22, 1980, the opinion of the FDA Cardiovascular and Renal Drugs Advisory Committee continued to be that the data was inconclusive. But on April 1, 1983, more than 3 years after the last official public discussion of the topic, and despite the availability since then of information from 4 further studies with negative results (Labarthe and O'Fallon 1980, Curb et al. 1982, Friedman 1983, Shapiro et al. 1984), the FDA required that "a precaution statement be included in professional labelling of reserpine (sic)-containing drugs stating that these drugs cause tumors in rats and mice" (Federal Register 1983). The only reference to epidemiological studies by this notice quoted the inconclusive summary statement from the Advisory Committee's meeting of June 1978, relying on "some uniformity across studies with respect to an association with 'recent use'". But time relationships were specifically looked for, and not found, by Friedman (1983).
Justifying this long-delayed and surprising action, a senior FDA official recently explained: "the decision had been pending for a long time and we had to do something."

Discussion

Case-control studies, although cheaper and faster than equivalent prospective trials, perhaps cost at least $ 500,000 each to execute to an adequate standard. The cost of the present series of studies is therefore unlikely to have been less than $ 12 million, or as much as half the total cost of development of a new drug. The suggestion advanced above that each may be considered as contributing one bit of information to the argument is manifestly absurd, but scarcely more so than haphazard and arbitrary decisions that apparently have little to do with the preceding well-informed discussions by experts in the field.

Any single study can be and usually is criticised, and so is exceedingly unlikely to be conclusive. There will thus be a need for a series of two or more studies, the results of which will have to be combined in some way. Several methods – of more sophistication than that proposed above – have been put forward, including simple combination of the probability values arising from tests of closely similar null hypotheses (Mantel and Haenszel 1959) to similar but more complex methods suggested by Jesdinsky (1984).

However, none of the studies and only one review have paid any attention to the intrinsic quality of the work. Henderson (1977) identified two aspects that caused her to consider that certain studies deserved more attention than others. These were the degree to which potential selection bias might have understimated the risk ratios, and to which potential exclusion bias might produce the reverse effect.

Hammond and Joyce had proposed in 1975 that relevant aspects of epidemiological studies of this nature should be exhaustively identified by a panel of expects (1975); that a second expert team should give a series of ratings to each study according to the extent to which it contained each kind of information in question; and that the resulting study profiles should be used to attain an over-all quantitative evaluation from the members of the first team. Many of the items, it should be noted, such as the size of the sample of cases and controls and of the population from which they were drawn are exact quantities; others, such as the adequacy of the methods used to acquire information on drug use or to confirm diagnoses, are scarcely controversial and can give rise to ordinal measures. The relative risk ratio, too, is a numerical quantity. The over-all judgment of quality might be multiplied by this ratio. The products resulting from succeeding studies could then be combined (a ratio of less than unity would be converted to its reciprocal and the product subtracted from, instead of added to, the total). The total quantity-quality product needed to provide sufficient conviction for justified regulatory action should be set in advance, in such a way that it could, in theory, be attained by a single paper. A sequential approach has been proposed by O'Neill and Anello (1978), but this solution, like all those previously put forward save that of Henderson (1977), does not take quality into account. Every one of us, including members of regulatory authorities and epidemiologists, does take quality into account when deciding how much importance to attach to our sources of information, both private and public. Lack of explicitness about the judgmental process unquestionably leads to inefficiency, and inconsistent and sometimes demonstrably incorrect decisions (Hogarth 1980).

But the original BCDSP "finding" was not wrong or a bad thing: a signal was obtained. The mistake was to present this signal as fact instead of investigating its validity. Cancer of the breast is an emotive disease; many women are depressive; hypertension and hence long-term reserpine medication is common in women; the dissemination of unproven conclusions of this sort has disastrous consequences and is hence irresponsible. All those concerned with evaluating drug side effects should be trained in ways of perceiving signals, to deal with them in a socially and scientifically responsible way.

Hulka, reviewing the similarly contrary evidence for a promoting (or protective) effect of oestrogens upon breast cancer, has recently enquired: "When is the evidence for no association sufficient?" She concludes that the most obvious way of resolving the inconsistencies is "to review the existing data with an objective eye and make prudent clinical judgments" (Hulka 1984). These aims can at last be given precise meaning. An experimental study of the epidemiological publications concerning the alleged rauwolfia breast cancer association, using the approach suggested by Hammond and Joyce (1975), is in progress.

Acknowledgments

Many friends and colleagues have helped to improve this account by their criticisms, especially Darwin Labarthe; and Oliver Pinto and the late Agamemnon Despopoulos, but they are not responsible for the deficiencies that remain. Teresa Harnisch typed several late drafts with good humour and great patience.

Summary

At least twenty-two further epidemiological studies (all but one published, the great majority *in extenso*) have investigated the association between breast cancer and previous use of rauwolfia alkaloids first alleged in 1974. Of these, the 2 published simultaneously with the hypothesis-generating study supported it but few of the others lent the hypothesis of an association any support. The great majority (18/23) of studies used retrospective case-control methodology, the known problems with which may have contributed to suggestions of an association. Some major sources of difficulty are pointed out. The results of long-term studies of carcinogenicity in animals have also been controversial. Nevertheless, some regulatory authorities have required warnings on labels and in package leaflets.

A causal relationship between the clinical use of rauwolfia alkaloids and appearance of breast cancer has not been demonstrated. Reserpine, the most widely used rauwolfia alkaloid, continues to be regarded in many countries as an effective and important antihypertensive agent. Its known clinical benefits far outweigh the harm from its alleged delayed effects.

Not only are the warnings inappropriate, but the rauwolfia case history throws into relief several important matters concerning the acquisition and evaluation of epidemiological data on adverse drug reactions that have general significance.

References

1. Armstrong B, Skegg D, White G, Doll R (1976) Rauwolfia derivatives and breast cancer in hypertensive women. Lancet II:8–12
2. Armstrong B, Stevens N, Doll R (1974) Retrospective study of the association between use of rauwolfia derivatives and breast cancer. Lancet II:672–675
3. Aromaa A, Hakama M, Hakulinen T, Saxen E, Teppo L, Idänpään-Heikkilä J (1976) Breast cancer and use of rauwolfia and other antihypertensive agents in hypertensive patients: a nation-wide case-control study in Finland. Internat J Cancer 18:727–738
4. Boston Collaborative Drug Surveillance Program (1974) Reserpine and breast cancer. Lancet II:669–671

5. Christopher LJ, Crooks J, Davidson JF, Erskine ZG, Gallon SC, Moir DC, Weir RD (1977) A multicentre study of rauwolfia derivatives and breast cancer. Eur J Clin Pharmacol 11:409–417
6. Curb JD, Hardy RD, Labarthe DR, Borhani NO, Taylor JO (1982) Reserpine and breast cancer in the Hypertension Detection and Follow-Up program. Hypertension 4:307–311
7. Department of Health, Education, and Welfare (1978) Report of the Ad Hoc Committee on Reserpine and Breast Cancer – Action Report (May 25, 1978). Washington DC, DHEW
8. Farber MD, Detels R (1977) Breast cancer and reserpine use in a population of hypertensive and normotensive women. Am J Epidemiol 106:238
9. Federal Register (1983) Professional labelling for reserpine drugs: revised labelling. 48:14048–14050
10. Friedman GD (1983) Rauwolfia and breast cancer: no relation found in long term users aged 50 and over. J Chron Dis 36:367–370
11. Hammond KR, Joyce CRB (1977) Psychological influences on human judgement, especially of adverse reactions. In: Drug Monitoring. Gross FH, Inman WHW (eds) pp 269–278 Academic Press, London
12. Heinonen OP, Shapiro S, Tuominen L, Turunen MI (1974) Reserpine use in relation to breast cancer. Lancet II:675–677
13. Henderson M (1977) Reserpine and breast cancer – a review. In: Colombo F, Shapiro S, Slone D, Tognoni G (eds) Epidemiological Evaluation of Drugs. Proceedings of the International Symposium on Epidemiological Evaluation of Drugs, Milan, 2–4 May, 1977 Amsterdam, Elsevier/North Holland Biomedical Press
14. Hogarth R (1980) Judgement and Choice. Wiley, Chichester
15. Hulka B (1984) When is the evidence for "no association" sufficient? JAMA 252:81–82
16. Hypertension Detection and Follow-up Program Cooperative Group (1979) Five year findings of the hypertension detection and follow-up program. Reduction in mortality of persons with high blood pressure, including mild hypertension. JAMA 242:2562–2571
17. International Agency for Research on Cancer (1980) Evaluation of the Carcinogenic Risk of Chemicals to Humans. IARC Monog 24:211–241
18. Jesdinsky HJ (1984) Pooling trial results. Society for Clinical trials 5th Annual Meeting, Miami, Florida, p 49
19. Jus A, Fabia J, Bernard P-M, Jus K (1976) Reserpine and breast cancer: a retrospective cohort study. Unpublished manuscript pp 12 (see also Jus A et al., Am J Psychiat 133:451–452)
20. Kewitz H, Jesdinsky HJ, Schröter P-M, Lindtner E (1977): Reserpine and breast cancer in women in Germany. Eur J Clin Pharmacol 11:79–83
21. Kodlin D, McCarthy N (1978) Reserpine and breast cancer. Cancer 41:761–768
22. Labarthe DR (1979) Methodologic variation in case-control studies of reserpine and breast cancer. J Chron Dis 32:95–104
23. Labarthe DR, O'Fallon WM (1980) A community-based longitudinal study of 2,000 hypertensive women. JAMA 243:2304–2310
24. Laska EM, Siegel C, Meisner M, Fischer S, Wanderling J (1975) Matched-pairs study of reserpine use and breast cancer. Lancet II:296–300
25. Lilienfeld AM, Chang L, Thomas DB, Levin ML (1975) Rauwolfia derivatives and breast cancer. Johns Hopkins Med J 139:41–50
26. Mack TM, Henderson BE, Gerkins VR, Arthur M, Baptista J, Pike MC (1975) Reserpine and breast cancer in a retirement community. New Engl J Med 292:1366–1371
27. Management Committee (1980) The Australian Therapeutic Trial in Mild Hypertension. Lancet I:1261–1267
28. Mantel N, Haenszel W (1959) Statistical aspects of the analysis of data from retrospective studies of disease. J Nat Cancer Inst 252:719–748
29. Miller ST, Runyan JW (1975) Absence of association between rauwolfia alkaloids and breast cancer. J Tenn Med Ass 68:657–658
30. Moriwaki S, Takashima S, Fukuda K (1978) Relationship between breast cancer and blood pressure as well as hypotensors. Clin Aspects Cancer 24:98–101
31. Moser M (1977) Report of the Joint National Committee on Detection, Evaluation and Treatment of High Blood Pressure: A Cooperative Study. JAMA 237:255–261
32. O'Fallon WM, Labarthe DR, Kurland LT (1975) A case-control study in Olmsted County, Minnesota. Lancet II:292–296

33. O'Neill RT, Anello C (1978) Case-control studies: a sequential approach. Am J Epidem 108:415
34. Shapiro S, Parsells JL, Rosenberg L, Kaufman DW, Stolley PD, Schottenfeld D (1984) Risk of breast cancer in relation to the use of rauwolfia alkaloids. Eur J Clin Pharmacol 26:143–146
35. Simpson FO (1975) Rauwolfia and breast cancer. NZ Med J 82:138
36. Takatani O, Kuno K, Yoshida Y, Terasawa T, Fujimori M (1978) Clinical epidemiological studies on reserpine use in relation to breast cancer among Japanese women. Proc Jap Cancer Ass 37:283
37. Veterans Administration Cooperative Study Group on Antihypertensive Agents (1977) Propranolol in the treatment of hypertension. JAMA 237:2303–2310
38. Watanuki T (1977) Analysis of answers to the questionnaire on breast cancer and reserpine. J Jap Soc Treat Cancer 12:123–124
39. Williams RR, Feinleib M, Connor RJ, Stegens NL (1978) Case-control study of antihypertensive and diuretic use by women with malignant and benign breast lesions detected in a mammography screening program. J Nat Cancer Inst 61:327–335

Author's address:
Dr. C.R.B. Joyce
Ciba-Geigy AG
Medical Department
CH-4002 Basel
Switzerland

Discussion

JOYCE:
There were no questions or comments following this speaker's presentation.

The organisation of long-term intervention and prevention studies

M. D. Rawlins

Introduction

Risk: benefit decision making lies at the heart of modern therapeutics, and it is possible to distinguish between four categories of problem.

Lethal disorders

Conditions which, in the short-term, have a high mortality can be readily subjected to risk: benefit analysis by conventional placebo or comparative clinical trials. Formal decision analysis can then be used to decide on appropriate therapy (Fischloff et al. 1981) and such methods have been widely adopted in the fields of oncology and infections diseases.

Chronic disabling diseases

Chronic disabling diseases such as rheumatoid arthritis, ankylosing spondylitis, major psychoses and multiple sclerosis, which tend to have a variable and fluctuating natural history, provide much greater problems in risk: benefit analysis. Although the short-term benefits of treatment may be easily demonstrated in patients suffering from more severe forms of the particular condition, in those with milder manifestations the balance between benefit and risk may be more difficult to assess. In resolving this dilemma, considerable reliance is placed on professional judgement which, despite its limitations, is the only solution we have to offer in our current state of ignorance.

Temporarily disabling conditions

Professional judgement is also used extensively in the risk: benefit assessment of treatments for self-limiting conditions such as soft tissue injuries, influenza, viral infections of the upper respiratory tract, migraine and traveller's diarrhoea.

Preventative treatment

Where drugs are to be given to prevent serious diseases, or the clinical and sociological consequences of both pathological and physiological processes, risk: benefit assessment has scientific, clinical and political consequences that cannot be resolved by conventional short-term clinical trials, or by professional judgement. Vaccination programmes, oral contraception, and active intervention to reduce the morbidity and mortality from arterial disease, congenital malformations or cancer, in large populations, require formal risk: benefit and cost: benefit analysis if professional and public acceptance is to be obtained. It is in these areas that long-term intervention studies have their most important role.

Construction

The construction of long-term intervention studies occurs at several levels. Arguably the most important is the *community* which ultimately pays for the studies and benefits from them. The necessity for a particular long-term intervention study must therefore be determined by the needs and priorities of the communities involved, and should be directed at their major public health problems. The *patients* likely to participate in a long-term intervention study also have an obvious stake in its construction, organisation and outcome. At a practical level their continuing loyalty and enthusiasm, based on a combination of enlightened self-interest and altruism, is essential if "follow-up" is to be accomplished over an adequate period of time. In particular, the mobility of patients in the developed world means that in the U.K., over a five year period, 40% of a cohort (especially if they are young) will have changed their doctor at least once. If their fate is to be properly documented, they will need to be traced using data banks that may conflict with contemporary anxieties over confidentiality.

Long-term intervention studies succeed or fail, however, mainly as a consequence of the quality, enthusiasm and persistance of individual *clinical trialists* who have the responsibility for recruiting patients, arranging the appropriate investigations, adhering faithfully to the agreed protocol, and obsessionally "following-up" defaulters. This degree of commitment requires that organisers of a trial take special care to involve trialists at the earliest possible stage; that they ensure individual problems are resolved rapidly; that there are regular and frequent progress meetings; and that there is an opportunity to meet and discuss the final report before it is published. The mobility of patients means that it may also be necessary to recruit secondary clinical trialists. These are doctors who were not involved in the study at its start, but with whom mobile patients have subsequently registered. Attempting to gain the interest, confidence and co-operation of these doctors is a very real challenge.

The *central organisation* of long-term intervention studies has usually been the over-all responsibility of a committee structure of varying complexity. The most successfull have been organised by national research agencies (e.g. Medical Research Council, National Institutes of Health), professional organisations (e.g. Royal College of General Practitioners) and independent charitable bodies. I do not regard government health departments or regulatory agencies as appropriate, for two reasons: first, the short duration of tenure of their personnel, coupled with their day-to-day pressures, are too great for reasonable continuity and consistency of effort; second, and perhaps more importantly, they have too close an involvement with other central government data banks to enjoy sufficient public confidence in the adequacy of personal data protection. Neither do I believe transnational pharmaceutical companies to be appropriate as central organisers of long-term intervention studies. Their interests in setting up the study may not be those of the community; they may be too closely identified with its outcome; and where there is dispute over the interpretation of the results, their impartiality may be questioned.

I do regard it as essential, however, that the day-to-day management of long-term intervention studies be in the hands of a single individual. Such a person is needed to recruit primary and then secondary trialists, maintain their interest, confidence and enthusiasm, sort out their individual problems, and act as a focus for the investigation as a whole. Dr. Clifford Kaye, who organised the Royal College of General Practitioners study on oral contraceptives, and Dr. Bill Miall who (until his recent retirement) was similarly responsible for the Medical Research Councils trial in mild-to-moderate hypertension, have provided exceptional examples of the dedicated commitment that is needed.

Finance

Long-term intervention studies are extremely expensive, and may cost anything from $ 5 to $ 20 million (at current prices) depending on their scale and complexity. In the past they have been financed by bodies such as the World Health Organisation, by transnational pharmaceutical companies, by government departments of defense and health, by national research agencies, and by wealthy charitable institutions. The source of funding for long- term intervention studies would be largely immaterial if it could be divorced from their central planning and execution. In reality, however, the scale of the investment that is required for such investigations makes this goal hopelessly naive since no organisation can afford to commit such large sums of money without the most careful scrutiny of the trial's objectives and design. As a general principal, the greater a sponsor's financial or commercial interest in the outcome of an intervention study, the more distant should be its relationship with its planning, organisation and control. In my own view, the preferred financial sponsors are bodies such as the World Health Organisation, government health departments and national research agencies, whilst the least appropriate are the transnational pharmaceutical companies. Ironically, recent history suggests that governmental organisations have been the least motivated to undertake the necessary financial investment. Regretably, I do not see this dilemma being resolved. Projections over the next ten years indicate that demographic changes and technological advances will result in an increased expenditure on health care which will be double that of the increase in the gross national product of most developed countries. This will place unprecedented demands on health care budgets, and whilst it might be logical to expect governments to respond by giving a high priority to measures aimed at formal risk: benefit and cost: benefit analysis, I fear that this will not occur. I believe that it is much more likely for governments to opt for short-term gains in other priority areas.

Neither does it seem likely that the pharmaceutical industry will find it any easier to indulge in long-term interaction studies. Development times of new chemical entities would appear to preclude the possibility that companies will contemplate an additional four to five years in demonstrating long-term efficacy and safety. I believe that it is more realistic, under current patent law, to expect the industry to demonstrate only short-term efficacy and safety.

Conclusions

It is possible to identify, with reasonable clarity, the organisational basis for long-term intervention studies. The primary problem lies in the source of their financial support. I doubt whether either government health departments, or regulatory authorities, or pharmaceutical companies, will find it possible to provide the necessary funds, and I believe that we must look to national research agencies and international bodies such as the World Health Organisation for a long-term commitment. We should therefore make strenuous efforts to persuade these organisations to deflect resources in support of long-term intervention studies. Unless we do so, the future of this important area of research over the next decade is questionable.

References

Fischloff B, Lichtenstein S, Slovic P, Derby SL, Keeney RL (1981) Acceptable Risk. Cambridge University Press, Cambridge

Author's address:
Dr. Michael D. Rawlins
Wolfson Unit of Pharmacology
The University
Newcastle upon Tyne NE1 7RU (U.K.)

Discussion

RAWLINS:
The discussion touched on three areas of the presentation.
First, the speaker's remarks concerning the inability of government to guarantee confidentiality of patient data and of industry to proceed impartially were challenged and some evidence for these statements was requested. In answer, the speaker restated his views in general terms.
Second, the question was raised whether large and costly primary prevention studies represent an efficient allocation of health resources. The speaker replied that where benefits or risks were potentially large this was clearly the case.
Third, a lively exchange of views ensued on the question of financial support for long-term intervention studies. Some agreement was reached that WHO itself lacked the necessary funds, but that this organization could play an important role in raising collaborative funds from member governments and from industry. The parasitic diseases program of WHO was put forward as a successful model for such a role.

The explanatory and pragmatic approaches in clinical trials

D. Schwartz and M. Pejovic

Some 40 years have passed since the introduction of scientific method into the evaluation of medical treatments, referred to as "controlled clinical trials"; in these 40 years the method has been in ever increasing use. Consequently, the question of the impact of its use on the progress of medical treatment arises. While a balance sheet would be difficult to establish, it is generally maintained that it has not been as satisfactory as it could have been, that many trials lead either to no conclusions or to conclusions which are not followed by results. The reasons for this state of affairs are many, but in our view one of the main, if not the main one, is bad formulation of the primary problem. This stems from the fact that the phrase "comparison of the two treatments A and B", contrary to appearances, is ambiguous and effectively covers two types of radically different problems, as can be demonstrated by examining successively two examples illustrating these two situations.

First example: trial of a new hypnotic

All controlled trials aim at *comparing* the *effects* of *treatments* on *patients,* so that the protocol must clearly define the four key words in italics. For the purpose of the present trial they are obviously and logically defined as follows:
1. *Treatments* to be compared: the test molecule and a placebo, the latter meant to create the conditions of comparison as "equal" as possible, so that the difference between the results can be attributed to the activity of the test molecule.
2. *Assessment criteria:* only a few, or only one if possible, to quantify the effectiveness, e.g. the duration of sleep in hours.
3. *Comparison* of the two groups: statistical test.
4. *Patients:* a sample chosen for reasons of expediency: ease of recruitment, sensitivity, etc., the question of representativity being considered of secondary importance: what is tested, in fact, is a very general biological property, probably capable of extrapolation from one population to another and the trial is thus an extension of animal experimentation. The above definitions are those routinely employed in present day clinical trials.

Second example: comparison of a new treatment (N) with a reference treatment (R) in rheumatoid arthritis

The aim of the trial is to find out which of the two treatments is "better" in practice, so that at the end of the trial either one or the other can be opted for. One can easily see that the four key words of the protocol can be here logically defined as follows:

1. *Treatments:* N and R for the two groups respectively, each under the optimum conditions: the optimum dose (equality of doses would be meaningless when dealing with different compounds), the optimum route of administration, with – possibly – secondary treatments and accompanying diet (sedatives, salt free diet, etc.). This definition completely disregards the "equality" of conditions as described in the first example. Such "equalization" could be achieved by giving, for example, in each group its treatment and a placebo of the other. However, this would introduce not only a complication but also an error, inasmuch as the trial is to be conducted under the actual conditions of use. Here, also, treatment administered blindly would not be justified.

2. *Assessment criteria:* these comprise a number of clinical and biological criteria pertaining to the condition of patients with rheumatoid arthritis and, in addition, the possible drawbacks of the treatments (their overall cost).

3. *Comparison* of the two groups: statistical testing is not an appropriate method for at least two reasons:

   – First of all, the null hypothesis "the two treatments are equivalent" has some meaning in the first example, inasmuch as whether a molecule is or is not effective is a scientific question which can be settled by testing; this is not true of the hypothesis "the two treatments are equivalent as regards the overall cost-benefit balance sheet". Not only is this question meaningless but the probability a priori is very low or even nil.

   – Secondly, in this example, the trial ends in a choice being made: which of the two treatments is to be preferred. Whereas with statistical testing non-conclusion is a possibility, in the case of our present problem it is but a façade, even a mistake, inasmuch as in the absence of a conclusion the doctors will continue to use the old treatment and thus arrive at a decision which is not necessarily the best. What is needed therefore, is the means for making a decision at the end of the trial and the best possible decision at that (in fact, in the appendix, we suggest a solution which has an advantage of simplicity).

4. *Patients:* This time it is essential to select a sample of patients as representative as possible of the population to which the conclusions of the trial shall apply; in effect, the result "N is better (or worse) than R" – unlike the biological property tested in the first example – is not a conclusion of general significance extrapolable to different populations.

Explanatory and pragmatic approaches

Whereas the two types of trials "compare two treatments A and B", it is obvious that they deal in fact with two entirely different problems. The first, which endeavours to test a biological hypothesis, has all the features of a laboratory experiment: selection of the most suitable group of subjects, an objective assessment criterion of – whenever possible – biological nature, treatments applied under identical and "laboratory" conditions, statistical tests to verify the hypothesis. The second, directed at choosing, in a given population, the better of the two treatments, is a kind of "general rehearsal", testing various treatments under real conditions. While the first type of trial is in fact a form of scientific inquiry and represents an attitude which can be termed "explana-

114

Table 1. "Key words" of the protocol in explanatory and pragmatic approaches

	Approach	
	Explanatory	Pragmatic
Treatments	Equal conditions	Optimum conditions
Criteria	Few, explanatory	Many (efficiency, cost)
Comparison	Statistical testing	Decision making
Patients	Selected group	Representative group

tory", the second aims at decision making, so that the approach it represents can be termed "pragmatic" (1). (The choice of the four key words of the protocol, representing the two approaches, is summarized in Table 1).

Error of approach

Definitions concerning the treatments, the criteria, the patients and the methods of comparison associated with the two approaches are so different that an error of approach in relation to any of the four key words renders the protocol inconsistent, so that the conclusions of the trial may be useless. This can be illustrated by an example taken from a field different than that of therapeutic trials but particularly striking. An agronomist, wanting to compare two strains of haricot, A and B, used an experimental design based on their growth in two adjacent plots. Strain A went all into the stem, strain B produced large clusters with the plants intertwined, interfering with each other's growth and obviously too crowded. Why? In a scientist's view an answer to this question would be provided by a test comparing the two strains under "equal conditions", i.e. with the same number of plants per sq. metre, how otherwise could one achieve "equality". However, this is not a scientific problem, inasmuch as the hypothesis A = B is meaningless. The problem is pragmatic: which one of the two strains is "better"? Once the pragmatic approach is adopted, the strains A and B must be compared under their respective optimum conditions (of density per sq. metre, soil fertilization, etc.); the conclusions of an experiment carried out under equal conditions would be useless.

Choice of approach

The two first examples selected as models of the two approaches and the last example borrowed from agriculture may suggest that the choice of approach is simple and comes to mind without hesitation. The reality is more complex and, in a majority of trials, the selection of every one of the key words is a "frustrating" operation, inasmuch as their advantages are associated with immediately evident disadvantages. A good example of this difficulty can be provided in a trial aimed at evaluation of acetylsalicylic acid (ASA) in prevention of postoperative thrombosis. These preventive trials, shelved for a long time, have been given a new impetus by the advent of the labelled

Table 2. "Key words" of the protocol in the explanatory and pragmatic approaches in a trial of acetylsalicylic acid (ASA) in prevention of postoperative embolism

	Approach	
	Explanatory	Pragmatic
Treatments	ASA/placebo*	ASA/low dose heparin
Criteria	Isotopic phlebitis	Pulmonary embolism and others
Patients	Surgery of the hip (high risk group)	Major surgery
Comparison	Statistical testing (comparison of incidence of isotopic phlebitis)	Decision making (overall assessment)

* If ethically acceptable.

fibrinogen test, whereby development of thrombosis is detected as local increase of radioactivity; this is a very sensitive test for subclinical thrombosis which in most cases does not proceed to clinical phlebitis: the lesion is termed "isotopic phlebitis". Table 2 shows in each of its two columns the possible choices for the four key words in an ASA trial. By examining the first column, the advantages and the drawbacks of the choice made may be summed up as follows:

Treatments: the only really strict method for finding an answer to the scientific questions "Is the treatment effective" involves the use (if ethically possible) of a placebo-treated control group. However, on a practical level the answer may be missed. This depends on the result observed: should the treatment prove ineffective, on the practical level the problem is solved; but further, should the treatment prove effective, is it also better than the orthodox treatment (heparin in low doses)? The choice of placebo control thus fits well with the "explanatory" but not with the "pragmatic" objective, the latter being achieved only if the recorded difference is not significant, an ambiguous result depending on the sample size. The same applies to the other key words considered below.

Criteria: detection of isotopic phlebitis represents a very sensitive criterion, as the lesion develops in almost 50% of cases, so that a small number of subjects may suffice. On the other hand, it is a biological criterion, "explanatory" as regards isotopic phlebitis and capable of solving the problem on a scientific level. However, on the practical level, the answer may be missed. This also depends on the result observed: should the treatment fail to reduce the incidence of isotopic phlebitis, it is probably ineffective and the practical problem is solved. On the other hand, should the incidence of isotopic phlebitis be reduced, does it also mean a reduction in the incidence of clinical phlebitis? This important question remains unanswered.

Patients: the use of a selected group of particularly sensitive subjects even if small but under good conditions should provide the answer to the scientific question: Is ASA effective? But the practical drawback is obvious: should the treatment prove ineffective in selected sensitive patients, it is probably useless, but should it prove effective in such a group, will it also be effective in unselected patients?

Method of comparison: statistical testing is suitable for the scientific-type question: is ASA effective? On the practical level, however, it is not satisfactory when decision making is involved; it may prove inconclusive, or the conclusion may provide no indication as to the ASA rating compared with the orthodox treatment.

Examination of the second column in Table 2 shows, for each key word, definitions whose advantages and disadvantages are opposite to those of the first column.

At every level of the protocol the choice is thus very difficult, simply because of the natural desire to include the advantages of both options. Clearly, the choices of column 1 provide for an answer to the question: "Is ASA capable of being effective in the form of prevention under study?", and those of column 2, to the question: "Is ASA better for this form of prevention than the orthodox treatment?" It would certainly be nice if the trial, long and costly as it is, could answer both these questions at the same time.

As, at the level of the four key words, every option presents advantages and disadvantages, as the choice is difficult, consistency becomes all important and one should not opt for the explanatory approach for some of the key words and for the pragmatic attitude in relation to the others. A logical sequence would be as follows:

– First comes the choice of approach. This is the problem of circumstances and one would imagine that, in general terms, a pathological condition would impose first of all explanatory trials, to be followed by pragmatic trials as several treatments become available (with a return to further explanatory trials when some treatments appear almost equivalent).
– Next, the four key words are defined depending on the option chosen.

For various reasons, notably ethical, this logical sequence is quite often impossible. A new molecule cannot be tested against placebo when a recognized effective treatment is already available. One may thus be drawn to a somewhat inconsistent protocol.

When the trial can be neither fully explanatory nor totally pragmatic, it is essential to recognize which of the two options takes precedence and to adhere to it as far as possible when formulating the protocol. This problem must be recognized by experts in clinical trials, as many inconsistent protocols are due to their ignorance of this distinction. The problem should be included in the teaching of trial methodology, with emphasis on what does and what does not constitute the distinction. This is not a prescription for easy protocol formulation but a tool for analysis and subject for reflection.

Generalization

The distinction between the two approaches, one aiming at knowledge and the other at decision making, greatly exceeds the framework of therapeutic trials.

In epidemiology, for instance, in the field of etiology, the distinction is very clear and can be illustrated by two examples. One is the famous piece of research on lung cancer, which first was directed at identifying the cause, then incriminated tobacco smoking and lastly endeavoured to prove the causal connection. The second example comes from perinatal pathology for high-risk pregnancy. Many factors allow us to predict an unfavourable outcome of pregnancy; using a few well chosen ones it becomes possible to identify high risk pregnancies and adopt measures unrelated to the risk factors themselves (more frequent antenatal examinations, choosing a well equipped maternity unit) which involves no investigation of causal connections.

117

The first example is that of scientific inquiry and the second is that of decision making. They illustrate well the two kinds of epidemiology, which could be qualified respectively as explanatory and pragmatic. As in the case of clinical trials, the two formulations involve radically different definitions as regards the four key words of the protocol, which in etiological studies are: the disease, the risk factors, the subjects and comparison of the groups.

Another example from epidemiology may be quoted to illustrate how the formulation of the problem may be clarified by the distinction between the explanatory and pragmatic approaches. This is also taken from perinatal pathology and concerns hypotrophic neonates, i.e. those of abnormally low birth weight (say, under 10th percentile, after allowing for gestational age). Certain teams are busy establishing tables or diagrams which, at best, provide a critical value for hypotrophy in function of gestational age. For this purpose, they produce different tables according to sex, parity and perhaps other factors, but the list of such factors may be shorter or longer and a number of questions arise: is it, for instance, necessary to include maternal tobacco smoking which is associated with low birth weight? One form of approach may be, obviously, explanatory, involving studies of factors influencing the birth weight, in which case the list should be as long as possible and should include maternal tobacco smoking; this approach would not require separation into two classes of birth weight. The other method of approach would relate to the decision making by a doctor who will have to undertake certain measures whenever the birth weight falls below a certain critical value; hence the need for distinguishing two classes, hypotrophic and "normal", separated by a critical weight value, and the problem becomes one of fixing this value in function of factors which justify a higher or lower birth weight: the sex is obviously one of them, while maternal smoking is certainly not; perhaps the height of the mother and of the father plays a role. The roles of the maternal weight and parity are doubtful. The problem merits discussion but one thing is certain; no advance will be made unless the problem is formulated as either one of advancing knowledge or of making decisions.

The choice between the two approaches, and the mental process involved in formulating the problem, is obviously not limited to biomedical research. An example from agriculture has already been given above. Many forms of research in various fields could not but benefit from this preceding development.

Appendix

A method of comparing two groups treated with A and B in the pragmatic approach

A solution is suggested here in which the explanatory and pragmatic attitudes become the two extremes of a general process (1). Comparison of two treatments comprises 3 eventualities (Table 3) and errors of 3 types: if $A = B$, but the conclusion is one of difference (risk of the first type, α); if $A \neq B$, with either no conclusion (risk of the second type, β), or with conclusion that the better treatment is worse, a risk which can be referred to as the third type, or γ.

In the explanatory approach one would like to test the hypothesis $A = B$, with the lowest possible values for α and β; obviously one would also like the value for γ to be low, but it can be shown that when α and β are low, γ is quite negligible, which is why

Table 3. Method of comparison of two treatments and types of error

Reality	Conclusion		
	B–A<0	B–A=0 No conclusion	B–A>0
B–A<0		Error type II β	Error type III γ
B–A=0	Error type I $\alpha/2$		Error type I $\alpha/2$
B–A>0	Error type III γ	Error type II β	

in the classical test of null hypothesis γ is always ignored; it suffices to select a number of patients which would guarantee that for a given risk α, the risk involved is in addition equal to the given value β, leaving out a given difference Δ.

In the pragmatic approach, the situation is entirely different. Should A = B, what would be the practical drawback of using A in preference to B, or of using B in preference to A, i.e. of concluding that a difference exists? In this case, there is no reason for wanting the value for α to be low, being of no importance; it can, in fact, be taken as high as possible, inasmuch as the higher it is, the lower is the number of subjects required. Therefore, let $\alpha = 100\%$. It is easily shown that in that case $\beta = 0\%$, which corresponds to the other requirement of the pragmatic approach: the risk of arriving at no conclusion will be nil, so that in any case a decision will be made. The only risk to establish is thus γ, which one would obviously want to be as low as possible; with this in mind one fixes the number of patients so that the risk is at the most equal to the given value γ of choosing the worst of the two treatments (the treatment inferior to the other by the given value Δ). Once the number of subjects is chosen on this basis, the conclusion of the trial will be achieved with a "degenerate" test at risk, $\alpha = 100\%$, $\beta = 0\%$, i.e. in fact, without a test: of the two treatments one adopts that which gives the better result.

In all these considerations we postulated a comparison between two groups with one variable x. In the explanatory approach, the variable x is – in principle – the only criterion adopted for the trial. In the pragmatic approach a complication arises from the introduction of multiple variables of efficiency and cost. Various methods may be envisaged for reducing the list, so that a single final variable is taken into account (1).

References

1. Schwartz D, Flamant R, Lellouch J (1970) L'Essais Thérapeutique chez l'Homme. Flammarion Médecine Sciences, Paris, and the English translation
Schwartz D, Flamant R, Lellouch J (1980) Clinical Trials. Translated by Healy MJR, Academic Press, London

Authors' addresses:
D. Schwartz
Statistical Research Unit
National Institute of Health and Medical Research
16 avenue Paul Vaillant Couturier
94807 Villejuif Cedex (France)

M. H. Pejovic
Department of Medical Statistics
Institut G. Roussy 94805 Villejuif (France)

Alternatives to classical randomized trials

Marvin Zelen

Introduction

One of the most important advances in modern experimental therapeutics is the development and widespread use of clinical trials to evaluate the benefit of therapy. The term "clinical trial" refers to a prospective clinical investigation in which the clinical investigator has control of the assignment of the therapy to the patient. A clinical trial can be contrasted with an observational study where one undertakes a retrospective record review in an attempt to determine the benefit of therapy which has been administered to patients. In general, the use of observational studies to establish the value of therapies is not reliable.

Of course there may be situations in which a therapy produces such a spectacular patient benefit that one can quickly come to a conclusion about the merits of a treatment. The use of penicillin is one such example. However, such extraordinary therapies are not common in the treatment of chronic diseases. Most of the time we are faced with examining a large variety of clinical situations where the expected gains are modest. One must recognize that a modest expected gain in the treatment of a chronic disease may have enormous impact if the disease is a common one. For example, it is estimated that approximately 27,000 women are incident with breast cancer every year in the Federal Republic of Germany. The median survival of breast cancer is six years. Hence an increase in the median survival of one year (16% gain) would result in an annual net gain of 27,000 person-years of additional survival for women in the Federal Republic.

It is of interest to contrast the differences between studies in medicine as contrasted to studies in surgery. The medical historian Bull (1) wrote:

"Whereas surgery made great progress in ancient times, the development of medical therapy was delayed until recent years. Part of this discrepancy can be attributed to the differences in the retrospective clinical trials demands. Much of surgery deals with lesions of simple etiology and often produces immediate spectacular results. Suturing of wounds and reduction of dislocations and fractures gives evidence of success at once and leaves little opportunity for elaborate theorizing. The fundamentals of such treatment had already been worked out in ancient Greece and Egypt. By contrast, few medical conditions could be understood until ancillary scientific methods had been developed ... It is thus not surprising that superstition and scholastic theorizing thrived and few therapeutic advances were made."

In order to cope with the difficult problems of evaluating the benefits of therapy for treating chronic diseases we have seen the development and rapid growth of an entirely new methodology devoted to placing clinical investigations on a modern scientific basis. The key to having credible clinical studies is to utilize randomization to allocate therapies to patients. The role of randomization in clinical investigations is sometimes not well understood by medical investigators who are accustomed to laboratory experiments where experiments can be repeated or discarded relatively easily. Also many physicians are used to relying completely on their own personal experience in the clinic for making therapeutic decisions about individual patients.

The role of randomization

The fundamental principle in comparing the treatment groups is that the groups must be alike in all important aspects that affect outcome and only differ in the therapy that each group receives. Otherwise differences in outcome between groups may not be due to the treatments under study, but could arise due to particular characteristics of one group not found in the other.

The idealized scientific experiment is where the treatment, which is to be applied to an experimental unit, is exactly reproducible from occasion to occasion and all experimental units are alike. This may be true in some areas of the physical sciences where the only variability encountered is due to the measuring instrument itself. Then the observed differences between groups are easily ascribed to differences between the treatments or methods under investigation provided the magnitude of the differences is not "obscured" by measurement errors.

However, in many areas of scientific investigation it is difficult or impossible to have homogeneous experimental units. Also the treatments cannot be exactly reproduced on every occasion. This is particularly true when the experimental units are patients who cannot be exactly alike and for whom a treatment may not be exactly reproducible. Consequently when one states that groups are comparable or alike, we mean "alike on the average" with respect to all factors likely to affect the principal end points. This characteristic of the different treatment groups being "alike on the average" is usually achieved by giving each patient the same opportunity of receiving any of the therapies under investigation. This is ordinarily accomplished by using a chance mechanism to allocate the treatments (therapies) to the experimental units (patients) so that neither the physician nor the patient knows in advance which therapy will be assigned. It is clear that one requires at least two therapy groups to carry out a randomized clinical trial. In our context, this means that the patient is assigned by a chance mechanism to one of the treatment groups. The major advantages of constructing treatment groups by randomization are listed below.

Advantages of randomization

It makes treatment groups "alike on the average" with respect to: prognostic factors, nontreatment related factors affecting the "drop-out" rate, and the censoring mechanism.

It eliminates conscious bias; e.g., physician selecting patient for trial, patient self-selection, etc.

It eliminates unconscious bias; e.g., unknown factors affecting treatment groups which may become known at the end of the trial or long after the trial is concluded.

It is necessary for validity of distribution-free statistical procedures. (This aspect will not be discussed here, but is included for completeness).

Among the reasons previously cited, the remark on censoring mechanisms requires further explanation. An observation on a time metric such as survival, time to re-

122

currence, etc., is said to be censored if the observation is incomplete. That is, a censored survival refers to an individual who is still alive at the time of analysis; in the case of time to recurrence an observation is censored if a recurrence still has to be observed. The censoring mechanism refers to the process by which observations are censored. Censoring always exists because patients enter a study sequentially in time and there has not been a sufficient follow-up period on all patients to have complete observations. When comparing groups, a bias is introduced if the censoring mechanisms associated with each group are not the same.

One must also keep in mind that there are some disadvantages to randomization. These are cited in the following.

Disadvantages of randomization

It interferes with the "physician-patient" relationship. The physician must inform the patient that treatment will be chosen by a random mechanism; i.e., "toss of a coin."

A patient or physician may not care to participate in a study in which the final treatment decision is made by a "toss of a coin."

A significant portion (usually half) of the resources may be expended in the control group. The interest is in a new treatment group. Many investigators desire to assign nearly all resources to the new treatment group.

New randomized designs

Despite the scientific advantages of randomization, many physicians are reluctant to enter patients into randomized trials because they feel it interferes with the physician-patient relationship. In the United States, the federal regulations (Title 45, Code of Federal Regulations, Part 46) require that patients give informed consent before being entered into a study by a physician. The informed consent procedure requires the treating physician to inform the patient about all risks and benefits associated with the trial, the alternate therapies available, and the patients' right to withdraw at any time. If the treatments are chosen by randomization, the patient must be so informed. Sometimes the randomization process is described to the patient as "tossing a coin" or "consulting a computer" in order to choose the patient's treatment. Randomized studies are not popular with many physicians. Some feel uncomfortable choosing a treatment by chance. Also patients, when informed of randomization, may decline to participate in the study and could even lose confidence in their physician. Ethically, if a physician has no preference or evidence to prefer one treatment to another, he should so inform the patient. Nevertheless, many physicians are reluctant to tell the patient he does not know the best treatment for the patient.

A recent survey by Taylor (3) among surgeons who chose not to enter patients on clinical trials found that 73% were concerned that the doctor-patient relationship would be affected by a randomized clinical trial; 22% disliked discussions of uncertainty with patients.

It is for reasons such as these that I published (4) a new way to carry out a randomized clinical trial which would not compromise the patient-physician relationship. These ex-

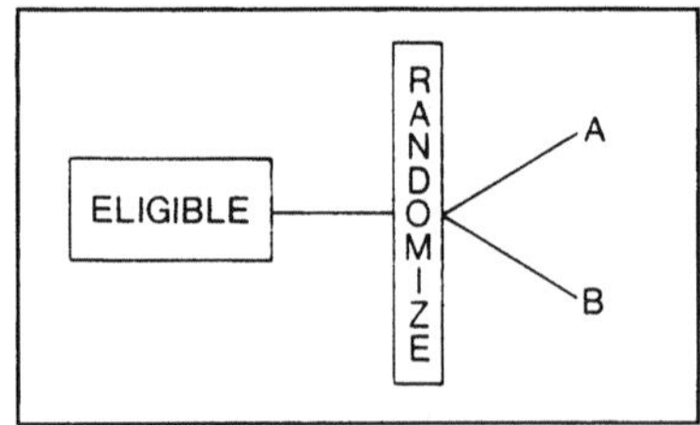

Fig. 1a. Experimental design from a conventional randomized study.

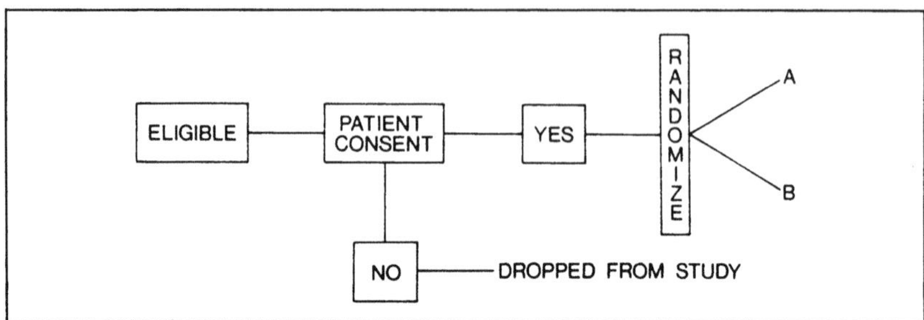

Fig. 1b. Experimental design from a randomized study with regard to patient consent.

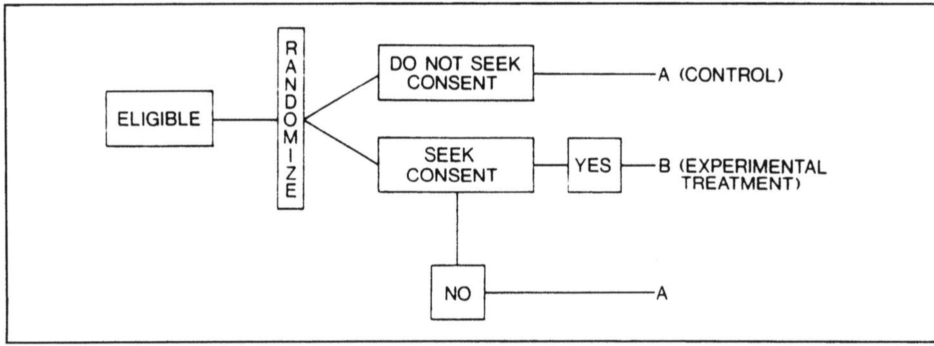

Fig. 2. A single consent randomized design. (A. Control treatment: Best standard treatment. – B. Experimental treatment).

perimental plans are called *pre-randomized* or *randomized consent* designs. This section discusses these designs. They will be considered in the context of multi-institution cooperative studies in which several institutions are pooling patients into a common study. Issues of stratification will not be discussed as this will detract from the main ideas.

These designs are put forth in situations where patient consent must be obtained whenever the treatment deviates from normal practice. In the U.S., the regulations are very specific about requiring consent whenever the patient would be at increased risk because of deviations from normal or standard practice.

The discussion will be simplified to include only a comparison of two treatments that will be designated A and B. Figure 1a shows the experimental design from a conven-

124

tional randomized study. Figure 1b shows the modification if patient consent is required. Even though physician and patient selection biases are present, the randomization equally distributes these biases (on the average) among the treatments.

Suppose that treatment A is the best standard treatment and B represents an experimental treatment. Treatment A is what a patient would expect to receive under normal circumstances. Figure 2 depicts the randomized consent design for this kind of trial. It is called a 'single consent randomized design'.

After the patient's eligibility is established, the patient is randomized into one of two groups. Patients randomized to the 'do not seek consent' group are not necessarily approached for consent to enter the clinical trial; they receive the best standard therapy (A). Patients assigned to the 'seek consent' group are asked if they wish to participate in the clinical trial and are willing to receive the experimental therapy B. All potential risks, benefits, and treatment options are explained. If the patient agrees, the experimental treatment (B) will be given; if the patient declines to receive the experimental treatment, the patient will (presumably) receive the best standard treatment (A).

The proposed new design has the desirable feature that the physician need approach the patient only to discuss a single therapy. The physician need not appear, in the eyes of the patient, not to know what he is doing and to be 'tossing a coin' to decide the treatment. Thus, the patient-physician relationship is not compromised. On the patient's side, there is also an important advantage; before providing consent the patient knows which treatment will be given. Many patients who agree to participate in a randomized study may have reservations about continuing after the treatment is known to them. At this point, some patients decline treatment and are considered 'cancelled patients'. However, others may continue the treatment, despite their reservations, because of the built-up momentum to do so and their reluctance to renege on their consent and possibly displease their physician. This design requires a decision by the patient only on the experimental treatment. Hence, the patient's decision-making processes should be more straightforward. This new design cannot be used when there are important reasons for conducting a 'double-blind' experiment, i.e., a trial in which neither the physician nor the patient knows the identity of the treatment during the course of treatment or its evaluation.

The analysis of this new design requires that group 1 (receiving only treatment A) be compared with group 2 (receiving treatment A or B). In other words, the comparison must be made with all patients in group 2, regardless of which treatment each received. Including all patients dilutes the measurable effect of treatment B. Nevertheless, all patients must be included if the analysis is to provide a valid comparison with treatment A. If only a small proportion of patients are willing to take treatment B, this experimental plan may be useless in evaluation of this treatment. However, the refusal of a large proportion of patients to agree to accept treatment B may be interpreted to indicate that it was premature to introduce the experimental therapy into a clinical trial.

Figure 3 depicts another kind of randomized consent design. We call this a 'double consent randomized design'. It is suitable for comparing two treatments in which there is no control or best standard treatment. Patients are randomized to each of the two treatments and then are asked if they wish to accept the randomized treatment. If they decline, they are given the alternate treatment or perhaps another treatment not under investigation in this study. Comparison of the two treatments is made by comparing groups 1 vs. 2 regardless of the treatment actually received.

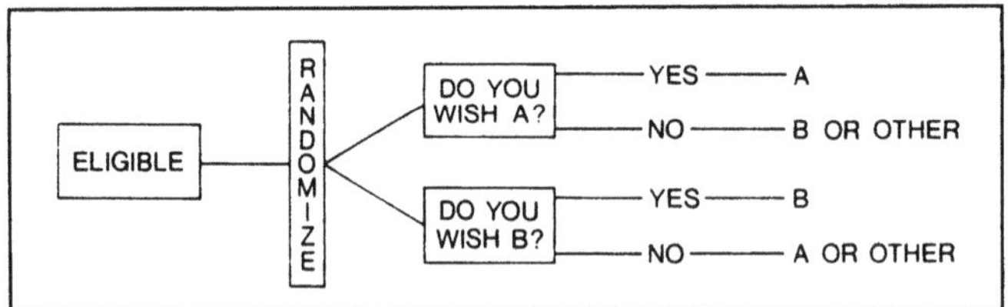

Fig. 3. A double consent randomized design.

Table 1. Efficiencies of single and double consent randomized designs

Probability of acceptance	Single consent		Double consent	
	Efficiency (%)	Break even accrual factor	Efficiency (%)	Break even accrual factor
0.50	25	4	0	–
0.60	36	2.8	4	25
0.70	49	2.0	16	6.2
0.80	64	1.6	36	2.8
0.90	81	1.2	64	1.6
0.95	90	1.1	81	1.2

Table 1 summarizes the efficiencies of the single and double consent randomized design. These efficiencies depend on the probability of acceptance of the designated treatment by the patient. For example, consider a single consent randomized design in which only 50% accept the experimental treatment. The efficiency of the design is 25%. This means that four times as many patients in this design are required to obtain the same sensitivity as a conventional randomized design. Thus, unless there is increased accrual by at least a factor of 4, this design may not be useful. The factor of 4 is called the 'break-even accrual factor' in Table 1.

Some ethicists have raised concern as to whether the single randomized consent design is ethical. The issue which has been raised is whether it is appropriate for a physician to enter a patient into a clinical trial without patient consent even though the patient is receiving best standard therapy. That is, there is no deviation from accepted practice and the patient is not at increased risk for being a participant in a clinical trial. Another point which has been raised is that the data generated by the patient on the best standard treatment will be used without the patient's consent. My own view on these matters is that it is the physician's choice to decide how to discuss matters with the patient assigned to the best standard treatment. Some physicians may wish to obtain patient consent – others may not. Either action may be justified. The use of the patient data from A in the analysis should present no problems. It is little different than a clinical department reviewing and analyzing its cases over a period of time in order to investigate trends in patient outcomes. However, most important is that the patient will know in advance if treatment will deviate from the norm and has an opportunity to decline the experimental treatment. In the classical randomized study, a patient gives consent prior to randomization but does not know which treatment will be allocated.

Recent experiments

Ellenberg (1984) has reported on recent experience with the use of the double consent randomized design. She reported on five major cancer clinical trials which used this design. Table 2 is adopted from her report. All of these studies were initially planned as conventional randomized studies. However, due to low patient accrual the experimental plan was changed to a double randomized consent design with the expectation that accrual would increase.

The introduction of the double randomized consent designs resulted in increased accrual for all five studies. However one must balance the increased accrual with the refusal rate of patients being offered a treatment from the pre-randomization process. In two of these studies (NSABP: adjuvant therapy for colon cancer; ECOG: adjuvant therapy for breast cancer) the increase in accrual was not enough to off-set the relatively high patient refusal rates.

It is instructive to examine the ECOG experience with a breast cancer study (1980) comparing adjuvant drug therapy to a control group for women receiving a mastectomy in which there was no nodal involvement (Stage I disease). The study was initiated as a conventional randomized design for 11.8 months and accrued at the rate of 3.8 patients/month. The study was then changed to a double consent pre-randomization and resulted in an accrual rate of 7.9 patients/month. However, due to an unexpected rejection rate of $35/124 = 0.28$, this experimental plan was stopped after 15.7 months, and conventional randomization was again adopted. The recent seven months of accrual shows a rate of 4.5 patients/month. It is worth noting that five hospitals had an aggregate rejection rate of $15/21 = 0.71$ during the double randomized consent period of the study. Questioning the investigators from institutions having high rejection rates indicated a lack of understanding of the double consent method. Some physicians decided in advance of registration the treatment they would use. Then the physician officially registered the patient and received a treatment assignment for the patient. If it was different than that which had been decided on, the "patient" refuses the treatment.

Table 2. Accrual and refusal rates in studies using prerandomization

Study*	Description	Date activated	Date pre-randomization started	Factor of increase in accrual	Refusal rate %	Total patients entered
NSABP	Curative surgery for breast cancer	4/76	6/78	6	11.3	1,742
NSABP	Adjuvant therapy for colon cancer	11/77	11/78	1.25	11.6	1,150
NSABP	Adjuvant therapy for rectal cancer	11/70	11/78	2	12.2	412
NCOG	Treatment of bladder cancer	3/80	11/81	4†	21	48
ECOG	Adjuvant therapy for breast cancer	5/81	7/82	1.75	28	170

* NSABP denotes the National Surgical Adjuvant Breast and Bowel Project, NCOG the Northern California Oncology Group, and ECOG the Eastern Cooperative Oncology Group.

It is for reasons such as this that one must be cautious in the use of the pre-randomized designs in the clinical setting. An essential preliminary before adopting these designs is to hold physicians' workshops to make certain that all participants understand how to correctly implement these designs.

The studies in Table 2 were all studies which were in difficulty with conventional randomization. Two cancer studies have been planned in which pre-randomization was used initially. One is a sarcoma study; the other is a melanoma study. Both are studies being carried out among several cooperative groups in the U.S. As of July 1, 1984, the sarcoma study has entered 10 patients with no refusals; the melanoma study has accrued 28 patients with six refusals. (Four of these refusals have come from a single institution.

Final remarks

The introduction of these new designs has raised new ethical problems about informed consent in clinical trials. Some of these have been discussed for the single consent randomized design. Another concern with these designs is that the physician might consciously or unconsciously attempt to influence the patient to accept the pre-randomized assignment. Actually this same problem arises in conventional randomized trials where the attending physician is attempting to influence a patient to enter a clinical trial. Perhaps another ethical concern, which is rarely mentioned, is the effect of the physician prescribing a therapy based on a poorly conducted study. One must weigh these consequences with the ethical issues of the physician attempting to enter patients on randomized studies using a pre-randomized design. The patient is approached for consent if the therapy is experimental (in the single randomized consent design) or if he/she is considering participating in a double consent randomized design. Unlike conventional randomized designs where consent is given by a patient to enter a trial without knowing in advance the treatment to be administered, the new designs discussed here enable the patient to know in advance of consent the treatment to be received. It is the view of this author that knowing in advance the treatment to be given in a randomized trial represents an advance for the patient. It is expected that over the next few years the use of these kinds of designs will be increasing.

References

1. Bull JP (1959) The historical development of clinical therapeutic trials. J Chron Dis 10:218–248
2. Ellenberg SS (1984) Randomization Designs in Comparative Clinical Trials. N Engl J Med 310:1404–1408
3. Taylor KM, Margolese RG, Saskolne CL (1984) Physicians' reasons for not entering eligible patients in a randomized clinical trial of surgery for breast cancer. N Engl J Med 301:1363–1367
4. Zelen M (1979) A new design for randomized clinical trials. N Engl J Med 300:1242–1245

Author's address:
Marvin Zelen, Ph.D.
Harvard School of Public Health
677 Huntington Avenue
Boston, Mass. 02115
U.S.A.

Discussion

Mr. Zelen's attention was drawn to the fact that when applying his trial design pattern the number of random samples will not be fixed any more, but will become random variables. He confirmed that this, in fact, is a problem with pre-randomisation and recommended that rules for the cessation of trials be set up before they are initiated so that trials will be stopped as soon as the given object is achieved. He also pointed out that for blind studies pre-randomisation is of no benefit nor would it make any sense.

When asked about the comparability of treatment groups, he explained that just as with the conventional design randomisation assures that the groups can be compared as to the mean; he admitted, however, that with small groups of patients with a variety of interfering factors homogeneity may be impossible to be achieved for each variable; for these cases he recommended an evaluation method that takes these differences into account.

In the course of the very lively discussion also problems relating to therapeutic studies in general were put forward that did not relate specifically to pre-randomisation. Zelen emphasized, for example, that a physicial preferring one therapy or another should not take part in a comparative study and, provided there is an individual preference for one treatment, the patient must receive this specific treatment and be excluded from the trial. Furthermore, he stressed the fact that a longer survival time must not necessarily be of advantage regarding life quality and criteria considering life quality should be seriously taken into account when setting up the trial design.

Data quality assurance with particular regard to protocol violations

O. Vanderbeke, R. Blomer

The collection of data is fundamental to clinical studies. These data contain the information which was the very reason for starting the whole project.

We all hope that this information will provide us with conclusive results. Only these justify the considerable effort and expense involved. These also, however, provide the only justification for our requiring the patient to put himself at the disposal of a project, which may well be of eventual benefit to society, but which at the same time may withhold from him the best treatment available at that time.

Data quality assurance has been described by Falter as the process which ensures that the contents of a scientific report reflect exactly the raw data collected.

This purely functional definition can be broadened to mean that data quality assurance should show that the report is indeed a record of what was originally planned, or what did not run according to plan. This widens the definition in the sense that it not only takes into account the actual dataset, but the whole course of the project, its planning and performance.

I would like to describe the approach we have chosen. It is only one example of many procedures which are possible.

Data quality assurance in this wider sense starts long before data collection. By that, I mean that the whole environment of data acquisition must be in harmony. The trial protocol must be unequivocal, the measurement procedures must be satisfactorily agreed upon and the case record forms should fit in with the routine of the investigator. Many a study has been unsuccessful because the case record forms – although ideally suited to electronic data processing – inexcusably neglected the investigator's situation. Above all, the number of variables should be kept to a minimum. Modern-day apparatus is, of course, extremely tempting, but what is not evaluated also does not need to be measured.

After data collection, i.e. usually after a case record form or specific parts thereof have been completed, the data collected should be immediately examined by a person well versed in such matters and involved in the study in question. The purpose of this is not to establish the absolute consistency of the data and their plausibility. Despite limitation, usually too many data are collected to do so. This should concentrate more on formal aspects such as legibility of text, missing data and whether the information provided for the principle variables is plausible. Outside the involvement of the computer, deficits in quality established at this early stage save much time and effort. This checking has the advantage of being immediate. Computer-aided procedures, even nowadays, are often still performed with considerable delay. Other projects with higher priority or at a more advanced stage are often the reason for this.

Technical data-quality assurance begins with data-entry. This means the 1:1 transcription of the written word into an electronically stored form.

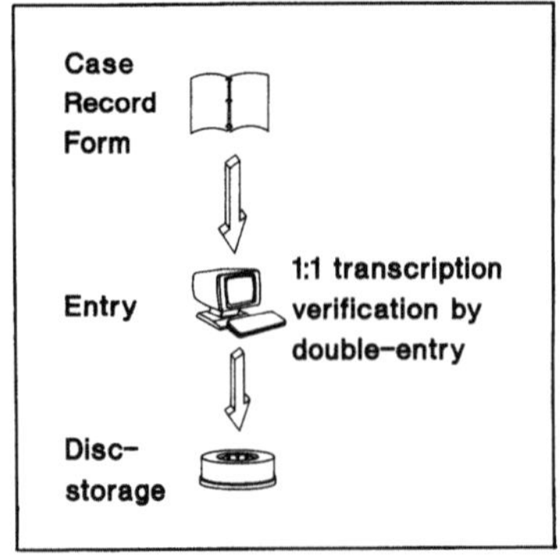

Fig. 1

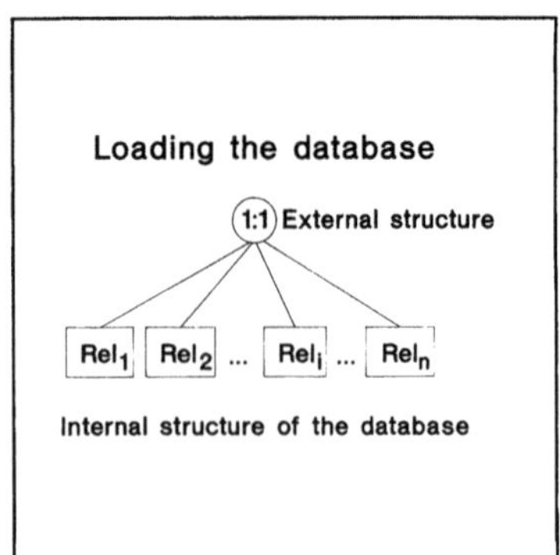

Fig. 2

It has often been discussed whether, and to what extent, data checking is appropriate at this point. This would be the very point at which the input of incorrect data into the computer could be avoided. I personally consider that this is not the right time to carry out extensive checking. The purpose of double-entry is to reduce the rate of input-errors. This is monitored by comparing characterwise a first input with a second input by a different person. More extensive checks disrupt the entry-person's working rhythm and inconsistencies found cannot be cleared up at this stage anyway, since it is necessary to contact several people, including the Medical Monitor. At present, remote data collection with the use of on-site microcomputers is being tried out in the USA. This means, of course, that data quality assurance might begin – if you like – at the patient's bedside. My experience with remote data collection goes back to 1977. At that time we tried introducing a so-called intelligent terminal into a hospital and the project failed. Perhaps the advent of the personal computer will raise acceptance.

The building up of a database (Fig. 2) follows entry which, as I have already said, is a 1:1 transcription. A data definition language (DDL) is used to model this database. Amongst other things, the DDL should allow exact description of the datatypes used. Our database uses the following datatypes:

Integer	Clock
Real	Time
Date	Code
Duration	Text

During transformation from the external to the internal structure, each datafield is checked for consistency with the respective datatype for this field. In this way, an integer field cannot contain any decimal points and a real field any letters. A variable of the type "date" must agree with one of the dates stored in the computer (Gregorian Calendar up to the year 2000). A variable of the type "clock" is only allowed a value of between 0 and 24.

A particular problem are the so-called code variables. Codes can be used to transform text into numerical terms.

We use, among others, the following codes:

1. ICD Code for diagnoses
2. WHO Drug Reference List for medications

132

Table 1. Examples for relations

Relation: patient demography

Inv	Pat	Age	Sex	Weight	Height
1	1	57	1	81	176
1	2	75	2	75	166

Relation: liver enzymes

Inv	Pat	Visit	Date	SGOT	SGPT
1	1	1	051083	12.7	15.1
1	1	2	121083	12.8	15.0
1	2	1	071083	15.1	14.9
1	2	2	141083	26.3	19.1

3. An extended version of COSTART, the adverse drug reaction terminology system developed by the FDA.

During loading of the database, each code is compared with those stored in lookup tables and codes which do not match are rejected. An error message is stored in the respective field instead.

Let me briefly mention the database model we have chosen – the relational model.

In a relational database, the data are stored in the form of matrixes, so-called tables or relations. Each column in these tables corresponds to an item – a so-called attribute – and each line to an observation unit. In these relations, one or more attributes must act as identifiers.

In clinical trials, for example, these are the investigator number, the patient number and, where applicable, the visit number (Table 1).

The data is stored in a clear and simple manner. Since there is neither a network nor a hierarchy, the relational database represents the absolute minimum necessary for later retrieval. Little conceptional structuring is needed while planning the database.

Consequently, changes such as adding or deleting columns or lines present no problems. However, the so-called data manipulation language (DML) for operating with relations must be very powerful.

DML is orientated on set theory. It allows for operations such as "union, intersection and difference".

Above all, the DML must enable interconnections between relations. For example, the joining of two relations to build a new relation needs relatively little programming (Table 2).

The introduction of new variables into a relation is equally as flexible (Table 3).

Our example shows a dichotomous variable which can be only "normal" or "high". This depends in this case on whether the SGOT is higher than a specific reference value (SGOTUP). After introduction of these variables all records where the variable is "high" can be printed out.

This is only a simple example for so-called range-checking which is part of consistency testing. Range limits are fixed for the various data before evaluation for the purposes of range-checking. As long as the data have values in these ranges, accuracy is assumed. If these ranges are exceeded, a printout is produced and passed on to the Medical Moni-

Table 2.

Patient demography			Liver enzymes		
Inv	Pat	Age . . .	Inv	Pat	Vis . . .
1	1	57	1	1	1
1	2	75	1	1	2
			1	2	2

Newrelation = Patient demography JOIN liver enzymes
        OVER
        Inv Pat
        KEEP
        Inv Pat Visit Date Sex SGOT

Newrelation

Inv	Pat	Visit	Date	Sex	SGOT
1	1	1	051083	1	12.7
1	1	2	121083	1	12.8
1	2	1	071083	2	15.1
1	2	2	141083	2	26.3

Table 3.

Newrelation

Inv	Pat	Visit	Date	Sex	SGOT
1	1	1	051083	1	12.7
1	1	2	121083	1	12.8
1	2	1	071083	2	15.1
1	2	2	141083	2	26.3

For Newrelation DEFINE

Newvariable = IF SGOT > SGOTUP
        THEN 'high'
        ELSE 'normal'

Newrelation

Inv	Pat	Visit	Date	Sex	SGOT	Newvariable
1	1	1	051083	1	12.7	normal
1	1	2	121083	1	12.8	normal
1	2	1	071083	2	15.1	normal
1	2	2	141083	2	26.3	high

tor for assessment. Examples of range checking are the reviewing of laboratory data as far as normal ranges are concerned and reviewing data for protocol violations. The standard ranges are, of course, also stored as lookup tables. The whole checking procedure is performed with a package of statements, compiled in the same way as the above example (Table 3). In addition to range-checking, logical relationships are also checked.

Logical checking means that data which are dependent on one another in some way are put into context. For example: the difference between two variables on subsequent visits should be no greater than a given percentage. If two data are functionally dependent on one another, the data should be distributed around a regression curve in a scatter plot. Points which do not do this must be checked. Incorrect data, which would not have become obvious in univariate analysis, can be discovered using multivariate procedures of this sort.

And, of course, multivariate procedures are not restricted to two-dimensional regression.

Let me now go more deeply into the sort of protocol violations we come across in clinical studies and the ways of correcting these which we feel are adequate.

First of all, however, I must just mention that protocol violations are the dread of all those evaluating clinical studies. They always leave a feeling of uncertainty in their wake, because there are no procedures to show whether the method used to compensate for them has introduced or reduced bias.

In my opinion, the most important protocol violations are:

Missing values

Missing variables

Dropouts/Withdrawals for unknown reasons

Examinations not following the schedule

Poor compliance

Changes in method of determination

Wrong diagnosis

Concomitant medication forbidden by protocol

Violation of randomisation

With regard to the way they are treated in the evaluation, they can be split broadly into the following categories:

1. Patients whose data can be supplemented by estimated values
2. Patients whose data must be excluded from the planned evaluation, but which can be used by applying additional procedures
3. Patients whose data may on no account be included in the evaluation

Cases where data are occasionally missing belong to the first category. Supplementary values can usually be estimated using appropriate statistical procedures. Introducing estimated values does, however, have its disadvantages. The number of degrees of freedom for the corresponding test statistic must be reduced by the number of estimated values.

The effect of changing methods of determination during a study can sometimes be corrected by transformation of the variables concerned. Here, every change has to be reported by the investigator. Changes which are not noticed can have a very disruptive influence – they increase variance and therefore also impair the sensitivity of the test.

Multiple examinations in a trial period for which only one visit was planned also belong under Category 1. In such cases, the following procedure is used:

The value obtained at the examination nearest to the planned visit is used in the efficacy evaluation. If side effects have been reported in this period, the most severe values are included.

As far as Category 2 is concerned, dropouts and patients withdrawn from treatment can usually not be included if variables are being evaluated over time.

In these cases, so-called endpoint analysis is carried out. This means that for all patients – including dropouts and withdrawals – the last value obtained while the patient was still being treated is used in the evaluation.

In a double-blind trial comparing two active substances, the number of dropouts may often be similar in both groups. In such cases, the conclusions drawn on both results will not be contradictory. The situation may be very different if the study is placebo-controlled. In such a case, lack of efficacy in the placebo group may result in many more dropouts than in the active substance group. It would therefore be worthless to carry out the evaluation as planned for the patients who completed the study, since this is a clear case of responder selection.

Patients admitted to the study with the wrong diagnosis and those who have received concomitant treatment which may have affected the results with the test substance must also be excluded from the evaluation of efficacy and fall therefore into Category 3. The findings in such patients must be reported on separately.

There are obviously still some cases which do not fit into the above categories. Amongst these are violations of randomisation. One of our standard checks is simply to sort the patients according to the date they were admitted to the study. If the trial has been carried out correctly, this check must result in a list of patient numbers in ascending order. Sometimes we discover that the investigator in charge of an open comparison has not kept to the randomisation plan. Instead, he has allotted the more severe cases to the substance he feels is more effective. This can result in a completely false baseline situation and lead to results which are not interpretable.

I think it is true to say that very many words have been literally wasted on the subject of poor compliance. Many methods to identify patients who do not comply well – and, in this way, to improve the quality of the data – have been developed and have failed, probably because the problem has not been taken seriously enough. Since this is a problem which concerns all pharmaceutical companies, I feel that the time has come to examine it in collaboration. I believe the best approach would be a research project carried out by specialists in the field to see how new microelectronic technologies can be applied to improve the problems presented by poor compliance – ideally backed by your association.

References

1. Assenzo J, Lamborn K (1981) Documenting the results of a study. In: Buncher R, Tsay J-Y (eds) Statistics in the pharmaceutical industry. Marcel Dekker Inc, New York and Basel, p 251–299
2. Falter K (1981) Data Quality Assurance. In: Buncher R, Tsay J-Y (eds) Statistics in the pharmaceutical industry. Marcel Dekker Inc, New York and Basel, p 301–326
3. Schlageter G, Stucky W (1977) Datenbanksysteme: Konzepte und Modelle. Teubner Studienbücher Informatik, Stuttgart
4. Wingert F (1979) Medizinische Informatik. BG Teubner, Stuttgart

Authors' address:
O. Vanderbeke
Hoechst AG
Klinische Forschung
Postfach 80 03 20
6230 Frankfurt
F.R.G.

Discussion

It was pointed out that even hard data – such as results of laboratory tests – cannot be compared in a multi-centre trial. Vanderbeke replied that efforts are under way to establish uniform measuring methods. For the achievement of an optimum comparability he referred to the possibility of establishing reference centres for the most important measuring methods and the application of mathematical balancing methods between the various clinical departments and laboratories, respectively, which as a matter of fact, are limited. However, he stated that there will still be variables that will have to be assessed directly in each clinical department involved.

Furthermore, it was emphasized that regarding data quality it is important to adapt questionnaires to clinical routine as far as possible; in addition, advantages and disadvantages of data collection in the clinical or statistical department, respectively, were detailed, but no recommendation could be given.

The need of clinical drug trials in children

D. Reinhardt

Introduction

Awareness of the age of the patient as a major determinant of drug efficacy has occurred largely through the dreadful drug disasters involving children among which the chloramphenicol-grey-syndrome and the thalidomide-phocomelie tragedy stand as only two examples. These adverse effects have prompted detailed pharmacological investigation which has shown that drug effects may be different at various developmental stages due to certain anatomical, physiological, biochemical and behavioral characteristics of different age groups of the pediatric population. However, although it is generally agreed that the solution to the safe and effective use of drugs is to base their prescription upon scientific data obtained for the drug under consideration, nevertheless with regard to the pediatric population the conception of the child as a "therapeutic orphan" is still too prevalent. Many factors may be responsible for this "therapeutic orphan" situation of the child and these include the ignorance and indifference of drug manufacturers and pediatricians, a negative public attitude towards clinical research in general and an uncertainty in the legal and ethical requirements for drug testing in children in particular.

This has led to the situation that for most drugs no dosage rules for children are available or that the drug instructions even contain disclaimer statings in the case of children.

I am far from demanding that pediatric studies be required for all drugs before giving approval for the marketing of a drug but it should be expected that pediatric studies be completed or underway for drugs tested already in adults that 1. have major advantages over drugs which have been formerly used for the same disease and that 2. could be used for treatment of diseases mainly occurring in children. There is no doubt that a complex interplay between clinical, ethical and legal aspects renders the task of studying the effects of drugs in children more difficult than in the case of adults.

However, because of qualitative and quantitative differences in pharmacokinetics and pharmacodynamics of drugs and the disease state arising from the different developmental stages of the fetus, the newborn, the infant and the child, drug studies are urgently needed before the drug can safely be administered to children.

Pharmacokinetics

The employment of adequate methods for the determination of drugs and their metabolites in body fluids, not to mention the great progress in computer technology, have made it possible to recognize the variations in pharmacokinetics between the different pediatric age groups and adults and also to monitor drug therapy under clinical conditions. Although variations in the pharmacokinetics of drugs may occur in each age group, most attention however has focused on the newborn infant. During the perinatal and neonatal period the organism is involved in a process of adaption and maturation which greatly influences drug absorption, distribution and the drug elimination process via metabolism and excretion (Table 1). Systematic studies concerning the age-dependency of a variety of drugs as for instance phenobarbital (Heimann, 1980) show an age-dependent acceleration of the drug absorption rate, but no age dependency of the total amount of drug absorbed. Since the bioavailability of a drug is determined by the amount as well as by the rate of enteral absorption this means that drugs administered to neonates by the oral route could have a reduced bioavailability as compared to the case of adults. In addition, the volume of distribution for drugs changes after birth. The protein binding is reduced in neonates and this may influence the plasma/tissue levels of drugs. The extracellular fluid volume, which constitutes the main part of the distribution volume, represents 45% of the body weight in neonates, but decreases continously with age and reaches 16 to 20% in older children and adults (Friis-Hansen, 1983). Since the body surface area corresponds closely to the extracellular space, drug recommendations should be made in relation to the body surface area.

In neonates, dosage calculations must consider the prolonged half-lives of most drugs attributable to impaired metabolic functions of the liver and renal elimination mechanisms. However although most drugs have prolonged half-lives there are exceptions to this (Table 2). Carbamazepin, phenylbutazon and phenytoin, although hydroxylated like other drugs with long half-lives in the neonate, show similar half-lives in both neonates and adults (Rane, 1980; Bartels, 1983), demonstrating that drug trials are a necessary line of research for each drug.

Because of the maturation process for some drug metabolizing enzymes other metabolic pathways may play a role as in adults. The best known example of such an alternative pathway of drug metabolism is the hepatic biotransformation of theophylline to caffeine via N 7 methylation in premature and mature newborns treated with theophylline for apnoic episodes (Bada et al., 1979). The methylation of theophylline has not been demonstrated in the normal adult human volunteer, where 1,3 dimethyluric acid (40%), 3 methylxanthine (36%) and 1 methyluric acid are the major metabolites (Fig. 1 according to Aranda, 1981). Thus research in the use of drugs ad-

Table 1. Pharmacokinetic peculiarities in newborns*.

Absorption	Motility decreased, acid production decreased
	Enzyme development delayed
	Bioavailability of many drugs altered
Distribution	Total body water increased
	Composition of the compartments altered
	Plasma protein decreased
	Binding capacity of albumin decreased
	Blood-brain barrier reduced
Metabolism	Enzyme activity reduced (maturation)
Excretion	Function of the glomerular and tubular apparatus reduced (maturation)

* Modified from Reinhardt and Richter [1981].

140

Table 2. Plasma half-lives (hours) in newborns and adults of drugs that are dependent on oxidation for their elimination*.

	Newborns (N)	Adults (A)	N/A
Aminopyrine	30– 40	2 – 4	>1
Amylobarbitone	17– 60	12 –27	>1
Bupivacaine	25	1.3	>1
Caffeine	95	4	>1
Carbamazepine	8– 28	21 –36	~1
Diazepam	25–100	15 –25	>1
Indomethacin	14– 20	2 –11	>1
Mepivacaine	8.7	3.2	>1
Nortriptyline	56	18 –22	>1
Meperidine	22	3 – 4	>1
Phenylbutazone	21– 34	12 –30	~1
Phenytoin	21	11 –29	~1
Theophylline	24– 36	3 – 9	>1
Tolbutamide	10– 40	4.4– 9	>1

* From Rane [1980].

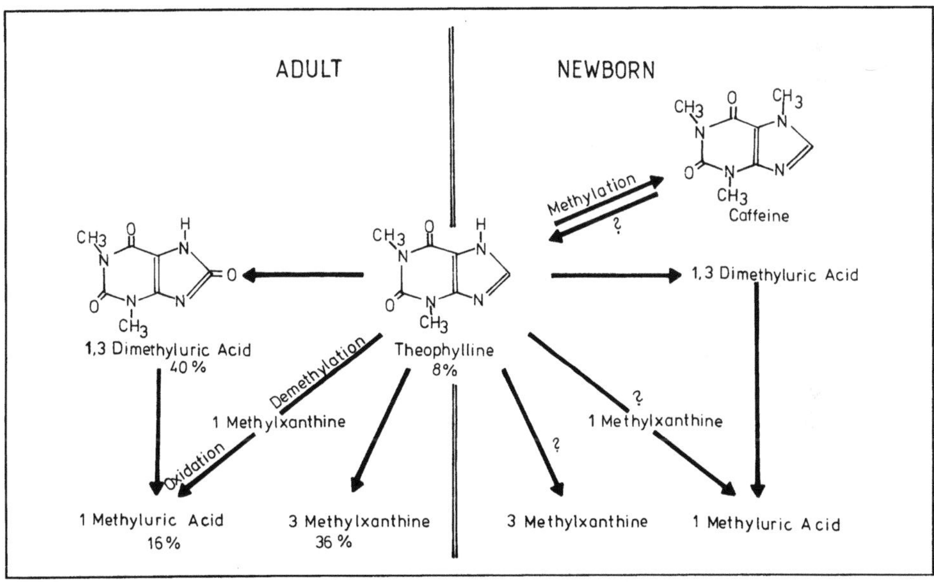

Fig. 1. Proposed metabolic pathways for theophylline in newborns and adults. (Adapted from Aranda et al., 1981).

ministered to children should include more extensive metabolic studies by far more than has been the case up to now. Although most attention has been focused on the newborn child, also in the older infant and child age-dependent processes may alter the efficacy of drugs. As Yaffe (1983) has stated "the maturation of an organism into an adult is successfully achieved only after the completion of series of intricate and interlocking events which proceed through a continuum". Theophylline elimination is known to be very slow in neonates and rapid in children beyond infancy, whereas within later childhood the rate of elimination decreases again (Nassif et al., 1981). As shown in Figure 2 the long half-lives for theophylline in the neonatal period decrease continuously until infancy, but were actually prolonged in older children and adults. Such a biphasic age-dependent aspect of a drug's elimination holds also for tobramycin (Pickering and Cleary, 1979), digoxin (Linday et al., 1981), some anticonvulsive (Bochner et al., 1978) and psychotropic drugs (Morselli et al., 1983). When age-specific dosage guidelines for theophylline were developed on the basis of the pharmacokinetics and on the assumption that the maximal and the minimal serum concentration during one dosing interval should lie within a therapeutic range of between 10 and 20 µg/ml, the biphasic course for age-adjusted dosages becomes evident and it appears clear that dosage requirements for neonates should be low, for older infants high and for older children lower again (Fig. 3 according to Richter et al., 1982).

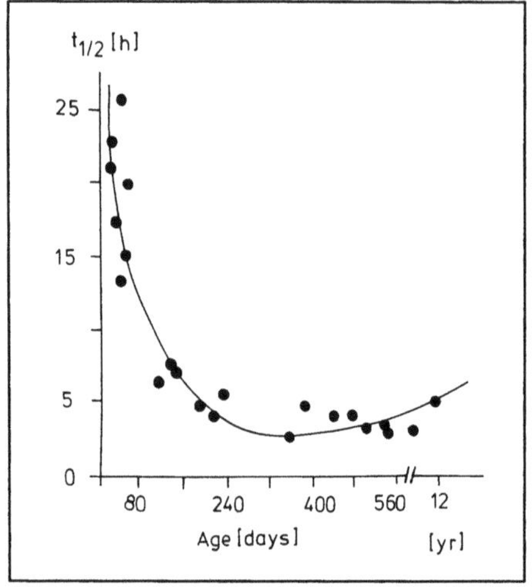

Fig. 2. Age-dependency of elimination half-lives for theophylline (according to own data and data adapted from the literature).

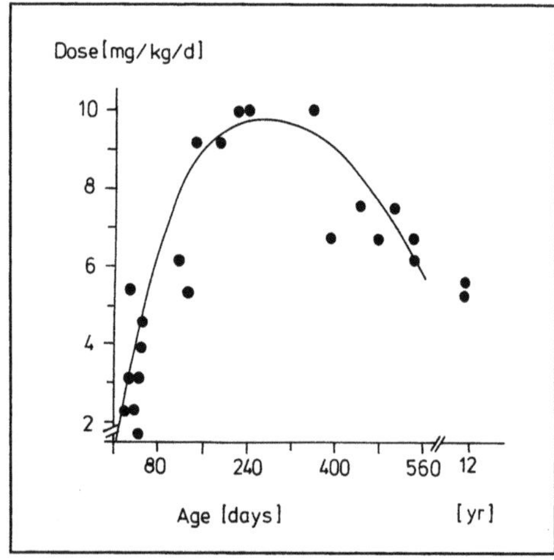

Fig. 3. Dosage calculations for theophylline on the basis of age-dependent pharmacokinetic parameters. It is presumend that peak and trough concentrations of theophylline should lie within a therapeutic range between 8 and 20 µg/ml. (for method see Richter and Reinhardt, 1982).

Pharmacodynamics

The development of new sensitive techniques for determination of drugs metabolites in body fluids as well as the great progress in computer technology have led to remarkable advances in pharmacokinetics in the low age range also and have even led to the practical assimilation of clinical pharmacology to pharmacokinetics. Pharmacokinetics however is of limited value for determination of clinical effects unless there exists a correlation between plasma levels and the drug effects in sick children. The problem of quantification of effects especially in the newborn often contrasts with the clear cut pharmacokinetic data. Boreus (1980) has illustrated the dilemma by evaluating pharmacodynamic parameters in newborns using the examples of pethidine, phenobarbital and aminoglycosides.

In my opinion apart from the restrictions on drug testing due to ethical considerations, pediatric pharmacology suffers especially from the lack of adequate methods of monitoring and evaluating clinical drug effects. Traditional animal models are not predictive and cannot be relied upon to supply answers regarding the effects of drugs during the timeframe of growth from conception to adulthood. Thus other methods should be sought in order to quantify pharmacodynamic effects. I will give you some examples. β-sympathomimetic drugs are largely ineffective in newborns and in infants suffering from an obstructive bronchitis up to the 18th month and as you can see from Figure 4 the bronchial resistance decreases only in older children in response to the β-sympathomimetic drug salbutamol (Lenney et al., 1978). It has been argued that in small infants a mucous swelling rather than a bronchospasm is involved in the bronchoobstruction. Others have suggested that the β-sympathomimetics could not work because of a poorly developed bronchial smooth muscle system.

In order to investigate whether a low number of β-adrenoceptors may account for the ineffectiveness of these drugs we have performed β-adrenoceptor binding studies with [125][I]-cyanopindolol on lymphocytes of a population which was divided into 4 different classes according to age. When binding studies on control and asthmatic subjects were analyzed by Scatchard plots, a clear cut age-dependency of the number of binding sites occurred, but there was no difference between control children and children suffering from bronchial obstruction (Fig. 5 according to Reinhardt et al., 1984). The K_D-values

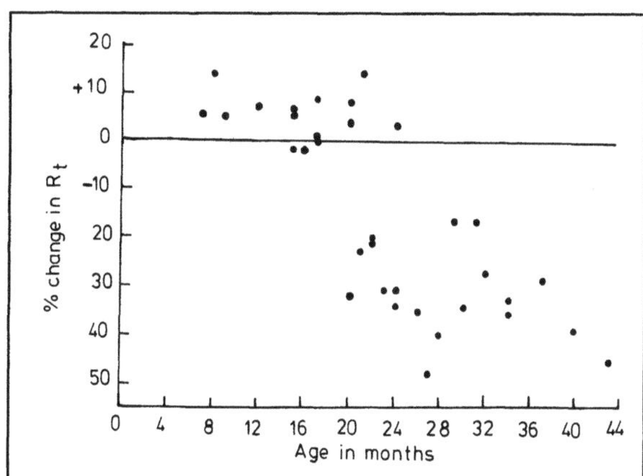

Fig. 4. Decrease of bronchial resistance in children suffering from a wheezy bronchitits after inhalation of nebulized salbutamol. (according to Lenney and Milner, 1978).

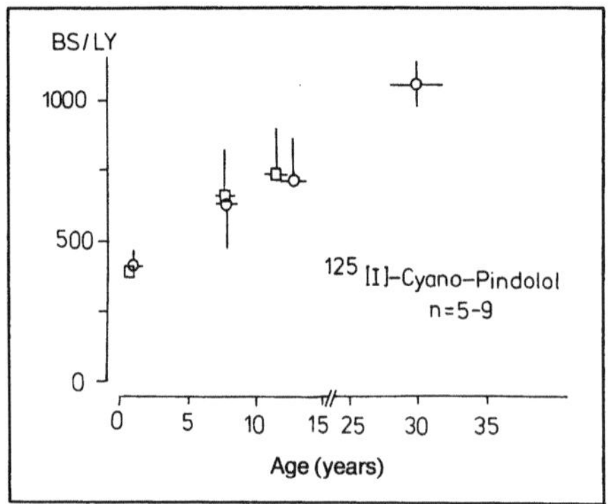

Fig. 5. Age-dependency of the β-adrenoceptor binding sites in lymphocytes from children suffering ($\square$) and not suffering ($\bigcirc$) from bronchial asthma. BS/Ly = binding sites per lymphocyte.

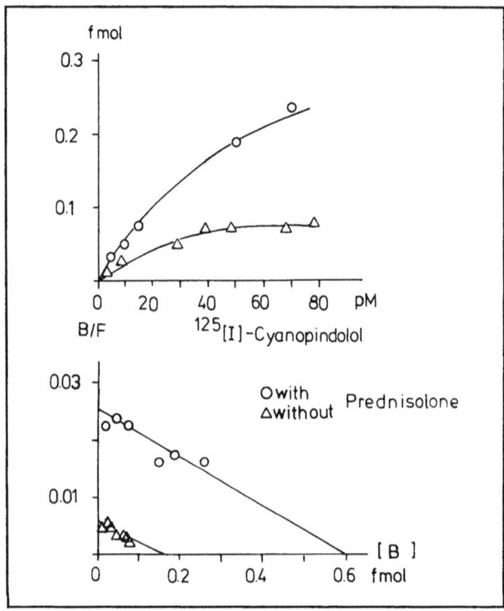

Fig. 6. Influence of prednisolone (3 mg/kg b.w. for more than 3 days) on the β-adrenoceptor binding sites of a small infant (3 mo) suffering from a wheezy bronchitis. Upper panel: binding curves; lower panel: Scatchard Plots. The number of binding sites per cell increased from 240 to 1644, whereas the K_D-values remained unchanged under prednisolone (according to Reinhardt et al., 1983).

showed no age-dependency. The number of binding sites per cell can be increased by the administration of prednisolone as in the case of the 3 month old infant who showed an increase of the binding capacity for ICYP after treatment with 3 mg/kg prednisolone which resulted in an increase of the binding sites from 240 to 1644 BS per cell (Fig. 6 Reinhardt et al., 1983). If this effect of glucocorticoids on blood cells is of any relevance one should expect that in the presence of glucocorticoids, β-sympathomimetics must work. That this is really the case is shown by Figure 7. The administration of the β-sympathomimetic drug terbutaline on its own does not reduce the bronchial resistance (empty circles) in small infants, but after prior treatment with prednisolone, terbutaline was capable of reducing the bronchial resistance (filled circles). This kind of experiment may show that (1) quantitative age-dependent differences exist also at the receptor level and (2) new techniques also allow the opening of the gate for pharmacodynamics. Nevertheless, differences in the anatomical tissue structure as well as a maturation of the endocrinological system may also affect the clinical drug response.

144

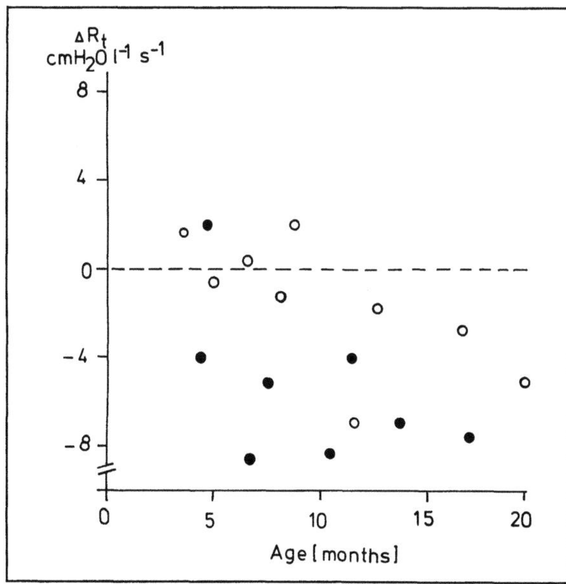

Fig. 7. Influence of terbutaline (0.3 mg/kg) on the bronchial resistance of wheezing infants before (○) and after (●) pretreatment with prednisolone. (according to Reinhardt, 1984).

Another concern that has arisen in the past decade within pediatrics is due to the greater interest in pediatric intensive care medicine. Low and very low birth weight infants who are often in a desperate situation receive a combination of a series of drugs which have not been previously evaluated before within this age group (Yaffe, 1983).

According to Aranda (1983) the very premature neonate has even three to four times greater drug exposure relative to the term newborn. Thus it appears to be not too astonishing that at least 30% of neonates in a neonatal care unit (Aranda, 1983) develop adverse side effects and the side effects may originate from the drug itself or from drug interactions. From these data it is clear that the occurrence of adverse drug effects in the neonate may even represent a major health care hazard, and it must be said that drugs in the neonate should be used with great caution. A safe use of drugs necessitates the availability of further representative pharmacological data relevant to the perinatal period, which data should meet the criteria of quality and validity.

New drugs

Awareness of the special situation of the perinatal organism, however, is a sufficient reason why new approaches to therapeutic intervention should be developed.

As a first example, theophylline has been widely and successfully used as an effective stimulant of the central nervous system for the therapy of premature neonatal apnoeic attacks. The reduction of apnoeas necessitates low dose recommendations varying from 2 to 4 mg every 12 hours. The desired plasma concentrations of theophylline to control apnoea without toxicity should be 5 to 15 µg/ml (Fig. 8 according to Myers et al., 1980). The narrower index relative to that for control of asthma in adults may be due to an

145

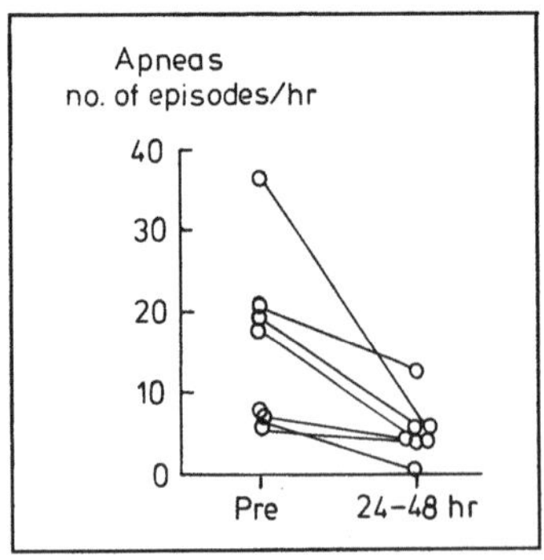

Fig. 8. Influence of a low-dose theophylline therapy on the frequency of apnea. (according to Myers et al., 1980).

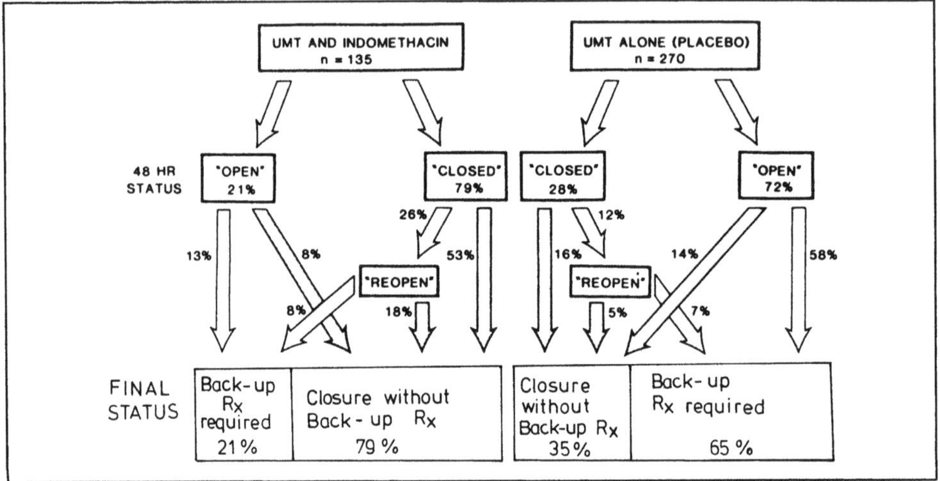

Fig. 9. Closure rates of patent ductus arteriosus under treatment with indomethacin and placebo according to a collaborative study. UMT, usual medical therapy; "open", criteria for significant PDA met; "closed", criteria no longer met; "reopen" criteria again met (Gersony et al., 1983).

additive effect of caffeine produced from theophylline in the neonatal period as it was mentioned before.

A further example may be the use of prostaglandines, especially PGE_1 which is now widely used for keeping the ductus arteriosus patent to maintain the pulmonary circulation in newborns with special congenital heart leasions. In contrast, indomethacin, a prostaglandin synthetase inhibitor, is used to produce pharmacological closture of the patent ductus arteriosus (Friedman et al., 1978; Heymann et al., 1976), which should it remain open is associated with an increased mortality and morbidity via a large left to right shunting.

According to a national collaborative study in the United States during a 48 hour treatment, 79% of the infants given indomethacin had no longer criteria for a PDA as compared with a 28% incidence rate in those infants receiving placebo (Fig. 9).

The reopening rate in the indomethacin group was 26%, but only 8% of those required a back-up treatment (by surgery). Thus the final closure ratio without back-up of indomethacin and placebo was 79% to 35%. This kind of treatment therefore renders a surgical ligation unnecessary (Gersony et al., 1983). The question of how early treatment of PDA with indomethacin would influence mortality and morbidity remains to be answered by careful clinical trials. The vulnerable phase of the perinatal period has necessitated not only a careful, strict set of criteria for the use of drugs and drug combinations, but also the research for new drugs for special diseases of this period.

In addition, one has to consider that the administration of drugs to the mother during pregnancy or the lactation period may influence the infant. A drug which has been intentionally administered to mothers for treatment of the fetus is dexamethasone. A double-blind collaborative randomized trial was initiated in the United States to evaluate dexamethasone as a method to prevent neonatal respiratory distress syndrome (Liggins and Howie, 1972), and there was evidence of a lower rate of incidence of RDS in infants whose mothers had been treated with steroids. I will not point to the calamities of drug experiments in which the fetus was made the inadvertent recipient of drugs administered to the mother. However there have been many examples in which epidemiological and pharmacokinetic investigations have yielded insight of how the fetus may handle the drug. The vulnerability of the fetus (thalidomide, diethylstilbestrol), of the very low and low birth weight infant and of the neonate (chloramphenicol, sulfonamides, oxygen) make it necessary that the sequence of drug testing in children should involve first older children then infants and then newborns.

Exceptions to this sequence may occur in the case of diseases which may be peculiar to one or the other age group. A number of special pediatric diseases in different age groups which require a special treatment could be mentioned.

The specific advances of cancer chemotherapy in childhood will serve as only *one* example of how well-planned and well monitored controlled clinical trials can give consideration to special treatment schemes for different tumors within different age groups. Clinical trials in the case of children with cancer are monitored by protocols of cooperative cancer groups. The individual procedure comprises the best conventional therapy combined with the testing procedure. An example for such a procedure (Tables 3 and 4) gives an intergroup Ewing's sarcoma study, in which all patients received radiation therapy to the primary lesion and were randomized to receive vincristine, actinomycin D and cyclophosphamide (VAC) plus adriamycin (Regimen I), VAC alone (Regimen II), or VAC and bilateral pulmonary irradiation (Regimen III). The continous disease-free survival following treatment was only slightly increased when a pulmonary irradiation was added, but markedly when adriamycin was combined with the standard protocol. The local control was achieved in 96% of the patients in Regimen I, and 86% of the patients in both Regimens II and III (Razek et al., 1980).

Table 3. Intergroup Ewing's sarcoma study (Razek et al., 1980).

Regimen I	VAC + Adria
Regimen II	VAC
Regimen III	VAC + bilateral pulmonary irradiation (1500 rad, 150 rad per fraction)

Each patient received a tumor dose of 4500–5500 rad to the whole bone followed by a boost dose of 1000 rad to any lesion with a 5 cm margin.

Table 4. Correlation of local control and NED survival with treatment regimens in 101 patients with comparable irradiation (according to Razek et al., 1980).

Regimen	Number of patients	Local control	NED survival[+]
I	34	33 (97%)	31 (91%)[++]
II	39	35 (90%)	17 (44%)
III	28	25 (89%)	15 (54%)
Total	101	93 (92%)	63 (62%)

NED = continuous disease-free survival following treatment.
[+] = Median duration of survival, 170 weeks.
[++] = Only 3 patients failed; 1 with local recurrence and 2 with distant metastases.

In future perhaps the in vivo comparison of drug combination will be completed by testing the drug effects in vitro on malignant and normal clonogenic cells which procedure may then in turn allow the tailoring of an individual chemotherapy to the individual patient. Although the therapy of cancer is crucial, the initial chance of cure for a child with cancer is often as high as 80 to 90 per cent and is thus far higher than in the case of adults.

Without aggressive clinical trials in the care of children with cancer the survival rate would be as small as 20 years ago and thus the tremendous advance in childhood cancer therapy may show how the rigorous evaluation of current treatment methods may be of benefit to the patient.

Final remarks

The essential guidelines concerning the clinical evaluation of drugs in infants and children should emphasize that the drug effects in children may vary from those seen in adults because of differences arising from the anatomical, physiological and biochemical development.

Although it should be taken into consideration that children, especially the neonates, are more vulnerable than older children, drug trials in all pediatric age groups are urgently required for those drugs which 1. have major advantages over drugs which have formerly been used for the same disease and 2. are relevant to diseases peculiar to special pediatric age groups.

Multicenter studies using uniform protocols similar to cancer study groups, as well as the new techniques to monitor pharmacokinetics and pharmacodynamics, will help to improve the unsatisfactory situation of the therapeutic orphan. Controlled and carefully made drug trials have a social function and if they had always been done under diligent surveillance the pediatric drug disasters would never have occurred.

It is necessary to emphasize this in our unsympathetic communities.

Reference

1. Aranda JV, Grondin P, Sasynink BJ (1981) Pharmacologic considerations in the therapy of neonatal apnea. Pediatr Clin North Amer 28:113–133
2. Aranda JV (1983) Factors associated with adverse drug reactions in the newborn. Pediatric Pharmacology 3:245–249

3. Bada HS, Khanna NN, Somani SM, Tin AA (1979) Interconversion of theophylline and caffeine in newborn infants. J Pediatr 94:993–995
4. Bartels H (1983) Drug therapy in childhood: What has been done and what has to be done? Pediatric Pharmacology 3:131–143
5. Bochner F, Carruthers G, Kampmann J, Steiner J (1978) Handbook of clinical pharmacology. 1st ed. Little, Brown and Company, Boston
6. Boreus LO (1980) Pharmacokinetics and clinical response. Eur J Clin Pharmacol 18:51–53
7. Friedman Z, Marks KH, Whitman V, Maisels MJ, Berman W Jr, Vessell ES (1978) Indomethacin disposition and indomethacin induced platelet dysfunction in premature infants. J Clin Pharmacol 18:272
8. Friis-Hansen B (1983) Water distribution in the fetus and newborn infant. In: Sedin G, Sjölin S (eds) Water and electrolyte balance in newborn infants. Acta Paediatr Scand, Suppl 305:7–11
9. Gersony Co M, Peckham GJ, Ellison RC, Miettinen OS, Nadas AS (1983) Effects of indomethacin in premature infants with patent ductus arteriosus: results of a national collaborative study. J Pediatr 102:895–906
10. Heimann G (1980) Enteral absorption in children. Eur J Clin Pharmacol 18:43–49
11. Heymann MA, Rudolph AM, Silverman NH (1976) Closure of the ductus arteriosus in premature infants by inhibition of prostaglandin synthesis. N Engl J Med 295:530
12. Lenney W, Milner AD (1978) At what age do bronchodilators work? Arch Dis Child 53:532–535
13. Liggins GC, Howie RN (1972) A controlled trial of antepartum glucocorticoids treatment for prevention of the respiratory distress syndrome in premature infants. Pediatrics 50:514
14. Linday LA, Engle MA, Reidenberg MM (1981) Maturation and renal digoxin clearance. Clin Pharmacol Ther 30:735–738
15. Morselli PL, Bianchetti G, Dugas M (1983) Therapeutic drug monitoring of psychotropic drugs in children. Pediatric Pharmacology 3:149–156
16. Myers TF, Milsap RL, Krauss AN, Auld PAM, Reidenberg MM (1980) Low-dose theophylline therapy in idiopathic apnoe of prematurity. J Pediatr 96:99–103
17. Nassif EG, Weinberger M, Thompson R, Huntley W (1981) The value of maintenance theophylline in steroid dependent asthma. N Engl J Med, 204:71
18. Pickering LK, Cleary TG (1979) Tobramycin dosage in children. Lancet I:102
19. Rane A (1980) Basic principles of drug disposition and action in infants and children. In: Yaffe (ed) Pediatric Pharmacology: Therapeutic Principles and Practice. Grune and Stratton, New York, London, Toronto, Sydney, San Francisco, pp 7–28
20. Razek A, Perez CA, Tefft M, Nesbitt M, Vietti T, Burgert EO, Kissane J, Pritchard DJ, Gehan EA (1980) Intergroup Ewing's sarcoma study. Cancer 46:516–521
21. Reinhardt D, Richter O (1981) Arzneimittelwirkungen auf das Neugeborene, Kleinkind und Schulkind. Fortsch Med 99:1551–1554
22. Reinhardt D, Becker B, Nagel-Hiemke M, Schiffer R, Zehmisch T (1983) Influence of beta-receptor agonists and glucocorticoids on alpha- and beta-adrenoceptors of isolated blood cells from asthmatic children. Pediatric Pharmacology 3:293–302
23. Reinhardt D, Zehmisch T, Becker B, Nagel-Hiemke M (1984) Age-dependency of alpha- and beta-adrenoceptors on thrombocytes and lymphocytes of asthmatic and non-asthmatic children. Eur J Pediatr 142:111–116
24. Reinhardt D (1984) Die Therapie der obstruktiven Säuglingsbronchitis. Monatsschr Kinderheilk. 132:448–453
25. Richter O, Reinhardt, D (1982) Methods for evaluating optimal dosage regimens and their application to theophylline. Int J Clin Pharmacol Ther Toxicol 20:564–575
26. Yaffe SJ (1983) Problems of drug testing in children in the United States. Pediatric Pharmacology 3:339–348

Author's address:
Prof. Dr. Dietrich Reinhardt
University Children's Hospital
Moorenstraße 5
4000 Düsseldorf
F.R.G.

Ethical restrictions in clinical trials in children

Lars O. Boréus

Controlled clinical trials of drugs are badly needed in children. The main reason why too few of them are made is the special ethical restrictions prevailing in pediatric research. Of course, methodological difficulties do exist, but experience shows that they can usually be overcome: the protocol can be especially designed for rapidly developing individuals and there are virtually unlimited possibilities to develop improved measuring techniques that are adequate for use in small children. These improvements may lessen the burden of risk and discomfort to the child and thereby make new types of pharmacological studies possible within the set ethical limits. These limits themselves, however, are not directly related to the progress in medical research. They are determined by public opinion in a given country at a given time and are not likely to change rapidly.

My starting point is one with which you will probably all agree: the clinical trial of drugs must follow the rules we have for clinical research in general. Among other things, this means that there must be a good scientific reason to perform the trial. The fact that commercial interests may be involved in the activity makes no difference. It is unfortunate that the reputation of clinical drug testing is still too often damaged by the appearance of poorly designed trials, or by trials that were never needed, from the point of view of the society. Drug testing for commercial purposes only must be considered unethical and should therefore not be carried out.

Ethical guidelines for clinical research may be found in The Helsinki Declaration in its original and revised versions. Also national Ethical Codes have been presented. The special problems in pediatrics are dealt with in codes issued by pediatric societies, for instance the British Paediatric Association. It published its "Guidelines to aid ethical committees considering research involving children" in 1980. Also, the Council for International Organisations of Medical Sciences (CIOMS) has, in cooperation with WHO, issued guidelines which include a section about research in children. The matter has also been rather extensively discussed in the medical literature and at international meetings. From this material relatively clear general rules have emerged for what can be allowed. However, to my mind, they are of little help when an Ethical Committee must take a stand in an individual case or in an individual project. They are very general and vague, as they must be, and should be. (The ethics of the interaction between the investigator and the drug company are certainly not dealt with although it is sometimes a "hot potato" in the media). They leave all the important decisions to you to make simply because these decisions must be based upon detailed knowledge of the patient's clinical situation.

Let us now consider the two most difficult and controversial issues in research on minors. These are to evaluate:

a) the balance between risk and benefit
b) informed consent.

Let us first consider "risk". There is general agreement that the risk for the individual child must be "minimal". It is up to the investigator and to the review committee to interpret the word "minimal". The British Paediatric Association, in its guidelines, defines three categories of "risk":

1. Negligible risk: Risk less than that run in everyday life.
2. Minimal risk: Risk questionably greater than negligible risk.
3. More than minimal risk.

The BPA states that "risk" involves physical disturbance, discomfort and pain, as well as psychological disturbance to the child or his parents. This is probably as far as we can go in trying to define "risk" in general terms; on the clinical level the determination of individual risk in drug trials requires thorough knowledge of the pharmacological profile of the drug, preferably including mechanism of action and pharmacokinetics, knowledge of the nature of the disease, and familiarity with the proposed techniques for measurement of effect. These are stern demands upon the investigator and almost by definiton they render Phase I studies impossible in children. Phase II trials may be performed, from the "risk" point of view, if data from adult patients speak in favor of minimal risk in children. This involves a translation problem from "adult" data to pediatric data. The dictionary for this difficult translation consists of our knowledge and skill in human developmental pharmacology. Past experience shows the devastating effects of unawareness in this field. A classical example is the Grey Baby Syndrome where cloramphenicol was given to term and preterm infants prophylactically in about the same doses per kg body weight as in adults. A cautious estimation will suggest that several hundreds of infants were killed by this exercise in ignorance. It was not realized that the capacity for glucuronide conjugation is very limited in new-born infants, especially in preterm babies, and that alternative routes for biotransformation and excretion of chloramphenicol are not able to take over. It is unrealistic to believe, in this way, that we would be safe by using simple dose reductions, based on body weight, body surface area, or age. It is also clear, from the last ten or fifteen years of research in developmental pharmacology, that studies in fetal and neonatal animals give little information about the pharmacokinetics in new-born infants. Predictions must be made from results in adults and in older children and the risk for the child is less if the biologically active metabolites are known in these older age groups. A monitoring system may be necessary to minimize the risk for accumulation of drug or drug metabolites. This may, on the other hand, sometimes increase the burden of discomfort or even risk, by means of extra blood sampling.

The burden may be lessened for the individual patient by use of non-invasive techniques. This is a more important issue in pediatrics than in other patient groups. In fact, the further development of developmental pharmacology in humans is very much dependent upon advances in non-invasive technology. Yoy will be able to do more within the set ethical limits. Yoy could also lessen the burden of risk and discomfort by designing the protocol in such a way that a trying interference, such as a venipuncture, a spinal tap, a respiratory measurement etc., is made only once in each patient. By means of careful planning, a time-effect curve may still be obtained. This possibility to reduce risk and discomfort is a potential but insufficiently explored possibility to make clinical trials also in "delicate" patient groups.

The notion of "therapeutic orphans" implies that the interest from the pharmaceutical industry to promote this area of clinical research is not overwhelming because the po-

152

tential market may be small. I hope that this is a misunderstanding on the part of more pessimistic colleagues; there is a need for improved drug therapy in many areas in pediatrics, both in industrialized and in developing countries.

The conception of "risk" cannot be grasped unless it is related to "benefit". In discussing "benefit" we immediately encounter the terms "non-therapeutic" and "therapeutic" research. In "non-therapeutic" research the results are of no benefit to the subject but may benefit the health and welfare of other children. The benefit may also be to add to basic biological knowledge; normal values for many functions are still poorly known for different age groups. "Therapeutic" research, on the other hand, is research that might benefit the actual subject of an experiment.

The difference between these two types of research has been the subject of intense discussion. Ramsey (1970) has argued that "non-therapeutic" research in children should not be allowed at all:

"A child is not to be made a mere subject in medical experimentation for the good to come".

The reason for this stand is that no one, parent or guardian, has the moral status to consent for a child to take part in an investigation solely for the gain of new knowledge. According to Ramsey, the moral progress of man is more important than the scientific.

A similar statement had been made earlier by the British Medical Research Council in their guidelines of 1963:

"In the strict view of the law, parents and guardians of minors cannot give consent on their behalf to any procedures which are of no particular benefit to them and which may cause some risk of harm".

This is an extreme standpoint which has been opposed by many pediatric investigators. It would effectively not only impede but also outlaw most research in pediatrics. Probably no new drugs could be introduced for use in children. Moreover, it would create uncertainty. At what age will it be possible for a child to determine whether or not to participate in a clinical trial? This question leads us to the core problem of informed consent.

The reason why we maintain so strongly the requirement of consent is respect for the autonomy of the individual. Autonomy means to be able to decide for oneself, to have the freedom to make choices. In this sense, the small infant has a very limited autonomy. He is totally dependent upon his parents or guardians and his freedom to make choices slowly grows at a pace which is determined by the parents and by society. As Cooke (1973) puts it: "We have graded autonomy – a graded freedom to choose". It is therefore logical that the parents or the family who exercise the autonomy should also be entrusted the task to give consent on the part of the child.

If we agree on the principle of proxy consent from the parents, we have certainly not solved all problems. If we have to deal with orphan babies with no parents to decide, non-therapeutic research, including drug trials, would probably not be approved in most countries.

Furthermore, family consent alone is no guarantee for proper protection of the child against unnecessary risk. How "informed" is "informed consent"? Can the parents really judge the risk or are they entirely dependent upon the doctor who informs them? The inherent information problem is sometimes formidable. In a recent application in our Ethical Committee the investigator wanted to take an extra blood sample and an extra pressure measurement during a complicated several hours long open heart surgery procedure. The increased risk for the patient was considered negligible and the protocol was approved. But how could the patient be informed about the nature of this small extra interference when the operation itself is never described to the patient on such a detailed level?

However, as far as phase III drugs trials are concerned, the information problem is usually not too difficult. Parents understand that without drug testing in patients improvements in therapy will hardly occur. What they want is assurance that their child would not suffer discomfort and risk. The combination of their trust in the doctor and the knowledge that the project will be reviewed by an independent expert committee is usually satisfactory to the family. In pediatrics, clinical trials often aim at an evaluation of already existing drug routines which have been introduced on the basis of empiricism. In our experience, this type of drug trial seldom brings difficult ethical problems as long as a non-treated control group is avoided. Randomization of the patients into different dose groups is one way to design such a protocol.

Internal control groups with non-treated patients are more difficult to set up in pediatrics than in adult medicine. Externally controlled trials make use of controls from another time period or clinical setting like in historical controls. Externally controlled studies must avoid many pitfalls but may, critically applied, give important and useful information. One example in pediatrics in the first reports on the successful use of indomethacine in persistent ductus arteriosus (PDA) in the new-born. They used only historical controls but were rapidly accepted; indomethacine has since remained the drug of choice for treatment of PDA.

A placebo group, or a placebo period, is usually permitted provided 1) that the child would not be likely to suffer more than minimal risk by being withheld from active treatment and 2) that the use of placebo is mentioned, in general terms, to the parents and, when possible, to the child.

According to the rules we try to follow for adults in our Ethical Committee, economic or other compensation for participation in clinical research should not be given to patients. Volunteers, however, will receive monetary compensation for pain and discomfort, as well as for travel and loss of income. If the same rules are applied in pediatrics, compensation cannot be given at all since healthy volunteers in the younger age groups do not exist.

A climate of confidence between the doctor, the parent and the child is necessary if an acceptable compliance to the given instructions should be achieved. Especially the prophylactic use of drugs involves great risk for non-compliance if the child is asymptomatic and if the parents have fears of side effects. A good example is the prophylactic use of phenobarbital against fever convulsions.

It may sometimes be a great advantage if the parents can be present during the measurement procedures. Openness is a basic rule. Be honest. The integrity of the investigator is the final resource.

References

1. British Medical Research Council (1964) Responsibility in investigations on human subjects. Br Med J 2:178
2. Cooke RE (1979) Ethical considerations in the selection and recruitment of children for research. In: Medical experimentation and the protection of human rights, N Howard-Jones and Z Bankowski (Eds). CIOMS, Geneva, p 165

3. Done AK (1964) Developmental pharmacology. Clin Pharmacol Ther 5:432–479
4. Proposed international guidelines for biomedical research involving human subjects (1982) CIOMS, Geneva
5. Ramsey P (1970) The patient as a person. Yale University Press, New Haven, p 12
6. Research involving children (1978) Federal Register 43: No 9
7. Working party on ethics of research in children (1980) Guidelines to aid ethical committees considering. Res Children. 1:229–231
8. World Medical Association (1972) Declaration of Helsinki. In: Katz J (ed) Experimentation with human beings. Russell Sage Foundation, p 312

Author's address:
Lars O. Boréus, M.D.
Department of Clinical Pharmacology
Karolinska Hospital
P.O. Box 60 500
S-10401 Stockholm
Sweden

155

Panel discussion:
clinical trials in children

Chairman: D. Reinhardt, Düsseldorf

Participants: L. O. Boréus, Stockholm
E. Deutsch, Göttingen
F. Seremi, Milan
H. W. Seyberth, Heidelberg
S. J. Yaffe, Maryland
D. Reinhardt, Düsseldorf

Introduction

Reinhardt opened the discussion with a quote from Franz Gross's introductory address at an international symposium on perinatal and paediatric aspects of clinical pharmacology in Heidelberg in 1980: "It is not exceptional that paediatricians consider clinical pharmacology an unnecessary line of research, a sub-specialty which satisfies the investigator rather than serve the patient. But this is not so. Careful studies with modern methods and techniques have to be undertaken in children and adults to make the best of medicines and in this way improve patients' care. These studies cannot be by-products of clinical medicine but have to be specially planned and performed to obtain results which permit valid conclusions. Clinical pharmacological investigations in fetuses, neonates and children are not performed to satisfy the investigator's curiosity or to improve his scientific image but have essentially a service function". Reinhardt then referred to the foregoing lectures on "The need of clinical drug trials in children" and "Ethical restrictions for clinical trials in children" from which had emerged that during the developmental period from conception to adulthood the spectrum of desirable and undesirable effects of drugs varies from age group to age group as a function of certain anatomic, biochemical and physiologic characteristics. In view of this fact, drug testing in children is indispensable. With regard to carrying out studies in paediatric collectives the question arises: What are valid scientific and ethical criteria? Over the last 15 years, pharmacokinetic investigations in particular have shown that, when establishing drug dosages, age-specific distribution and elimination patterns must be taken into account. As yet, however, only a limited number of studies exist on pharmaco-dynamics as a function of age. This is because – despite advanced technological methods – the action of drugs, particularly in children, is difficult to objectify. Moreover, there are many medications for which a correlation between plasma concentration and clinical efficacy has not been demonstrated or does not exist. Above and beyond these issues, the fact that, in childhood, other types of disease and courses of disease occur, necessitates the development of specific paediatric preparations. For all of the above-mentioned factors it is valid to say that the younger the child the greater the differences with respect to adulthood. Reinhardt then called attention to a third and equally important point with regard to drug testing in children, namely the special situation in terms of legal and ethical problems.

Special Aspects of Demonstrating Drug Efficacy in Children

Reinhardt questioned Boréus about the possibilities for and special aspects of recording and monitoring drug treatment in children.

In his response, Boréus pointed out that pharmacokinetic studies have revealed very fruitful methods of drug surveillance by means of therapeutic drug monitoring at least for a number of medications in children as well. However, since clinical observations have shown that children react differently from adults to quite a few drugs, future studies should also concentrate on pharmacodynamics in childhood. Boréus illustrated the necessity for this with several examples from the group of anticonvulsants. Phenobarbital, for example, is one of the most frequently used drugs in paediatrics. Despite the fact that its range of indications has recently been expanded to include cerebral haemorrhage in children, its principal indication is in the treatment of cerebral convulsions. A sedative effect, such as is observed in older children and adults, is difficult to demonstrate in newborns, since as a rule they sleep 16–18 hours per day. However, non-invasive methods for determining the action of the drug are available. By means of several hours of time-lapse filming of the child's movements it has been shown that the percentage of time spent in deep sleep increases in accordance with the phenobarbital dose. In general, a 6-year-old child given the same dosages would initially exhibit hyperactivity and restlessness, an age-related phenomenon familiar to all parents from their own children when overtired. The observed restlessness and hyperactivity in children under the effect of phenobarbital cannot be attributed to underdosage, since this phenomenon is enhanced with increasing dosages. Children between the ages of about 6 months and 5 years often develop, with increasing body temperature, what are known as febrile convulsions, something which has not been observed in adults. In approximately 80–90% of cases these febrile convulsions can be aborted with benzodiazepine. Thus, treatment of the acute symptoms is essentially non-problematic. Both phenobarbital and valproic acid are efficacious in preventing recurrent febrile convulsions. In contrast, carbamazepine and phenytoin, effective prophylactic agents in cerebral convulsions in adults, are virtually ineffective in the prophylaxis of febrile convulsions. This finding indicates that the response of the brain to different pharmacologic substances varies according to developmental stage. Boréus noted that glomerular filtration as well as renal tubular reabsorption and filtration also undergo a similar maturation process. For the various mechanisms of renal elimination maturation is temporally unrelated. This means that the effect of a drug can change in the course of a few days, depending on its route of elimination.

Reinhardt took up the example of phenobarbital to call attention to the fact that, in the context of specific paediatric diseases, new indications may be ascribed to long-recognized substances. Phenobarbital is thus said to be a meaningful form of prophylactic treatment in asphyxia and intracranial haemorrhage of the newborn. Reinhardt asked Seyberth if he could cite additional examples of the development of special drug applications in paediatric illnesses.

Specific Childhood Diseases

Seyberth answered that phenobarbital was probably not the best of examples, since controlled studies had shown that its use in premature and full-term infants to prevent cerebral haemorrhage produces more adverse effects than desirable effects; this has, however, done nothing to prevent its continued use at high doses for the cited indications. He mentioned treatment of patent ductus arteriosus as a typical example of the unique features of paediatric therapy. Formerly, based on experience in adult medicine, premature and fullterm neonates with patent ductus arteriosus were treated similarly to patients with heart failure, i.e., they received digitalis glycosides and furosemide and fluid intake was restricted. It was subsequently demonstrated, however, that digitalis glycosides were not very effective in newborns with patent ductus. Moreover, as a result of interactions with other endogenous and exogenous substances, drug monitoring by means of plasma level determinations was often impossible. Symptoms of overdigitalization were observed in many children. Renal problems occurred due to limited fluid intake. The administration of furosemide, often at overdose levels, caused sodium loss and additional renal problems. Further sequelae of therapy were hypercalcuria and nephrocalcinosis. In fact, due to stimulation of prostaglandin synthesis, an effect counter to the desired therapeutic effect was achieved. These findings illustrated that knowledge gleaned from adult medicine could not be directly applied to treatment of childhood disorders. In 1976 Friedman et al. (N Engl J Med 295:526) submitted the first report on closure of the ductus with indomethacin therapy. Since then, indomethacin, a recognized antiphlogistic and antirheumatic agent, has been used worldwide to treat patent ductus arteriosus of the preterm and full-term newborn. The results of numerous studies indicate that in approximately 50–70% of the children one treatment cycle with indomethacin is sufficient to close the ductus. Drug monitoring via mass spectrometry and non-invasive determination of ductal shunt volumes with the aid of Doppler sonography have permitted the establishment of dosage guidelines for indomethacin in the treatment of patent ductus arteriosus; this has increased the success rate to nearly 90%. Seyberth stressed the necessity for new drug principles in the treatment of other disorders also specific to childhood. He referred to the inadequate therapeutic possibilities in cerebral haemorrhage of the premature infant and the as yet insufficient treatment methods for pulmonary hypertension, where oxygen administration causes a further increase in pressure and tolazoline therapy produces a broad range of side effects. Seyberth also mentioned bronchopulmonary dysplasia ("ventilator lung"), which occurs in a high percentage of premature babies as a result of mechanical ventilation and causes a hyper-reactivity of the bronchial system – which can manifest similarly to bronchial asthma – even long after mechanical ventilation has been discontinued. The special situation of premature and full-term infants and the disorders peculiar to this age group thus require valid clinical pharmacologic studies in this paediatric collective. The examples presented demonstrate that uncontrolled use of adult-tested drugs in children is unacceptable. Seyberth referred to his own study on the intensive care unit of the University of Heidelberg Paediatric Clinic. Of 41 preparations used there in paediatric intensive care, investigations in preterm and full-term neonates had only been carried out for 5 preparations – and these were almost exclusively antibiotics. In small children only about 1/3, and in school-age children 1/2 of the drugs used had been tested in pharmacologic studies. In Seyberth's opinion, the situation with respect to paediatric drug therapy is further aggravated by the non-availability of suitable presentations for children; this is also true of drugs which have already been tested in children, such as digitalis, phenobarbital and theophylline.

Yaffe recalled to mind that a few years ago at a WHO symposium in Schlangenbad Franz Gross had stressed the necessity for cooperation between drug approval authorities, industry and university researchers. In the interim, however, little has been done to implement this suggestion and most of the drugs available on the market are produced and distributed for purely commercial reasons. Although he did not challenge the manufacturers' profit motive, he posed the question of how to convince pharmaceutical firms that clinical trials in children – even when commercially uninteresting – must be carried out. In Yaffe's opinion, the necessary technical equipment and personnel are available for such studies. He warned against assuming that differences in pharmacokinetics and pharmacodynamics are confined exclusively to the preterm and full-term neonate group. Also in other age groups, such as small children, school-age children and adolescents as well, anatomic, biochemical and physiologic changes are taking place which can influence drug efficacy. In the United States – similar to the therapy studies on paediatric oncologic diseases – a prospective and probably randomized study, including control populations, on paediatric intensive care units, on the therapy of various disorders of the newborn, subsidized by the National Institutes of Health, is being planned and will be carried out in the near future. Until now, the thought pattern which has prevailed in neonatology has been based on purely pragmatic principles, such as "the child has oedema; we must therefore administer a diuretic". The attending neonatologist is certainly not aware that no clinicopharmacologic data exist for oedema therapy. In the US, prospective studies on therapy in pregnant women are also in the planning stages. To date, there is a scarcity of information on what substances are both effective and safe for the pregnant woman and not harmful to the foetus.

Toxic Drug Effects in Children

Sereni pointed out that also undesirable effects of drugs are age-related. The common belief that a substance is all the more toxic the younger the child is, is not always true. It has been demonstrated, for example, that the nephrotoxic effect of aminoglycoside antibiotics, which are used in paediatrics to treat sepsis caused by gram-negative bacteria, is less pronounced in premature and full-term newborns than in older children. This is also the case at plasma levels higher than normal adult levels. From pharmacokinetic studies we know that the distribution volumes of aminoglycosides in very young children differ from those in older children and adults, also due to different tissue concentrations in the renal cortex and inner ear. In order to prove this, however, elaborate wash-out studies involving numerous blood tests and urinalyses are necessary. Tissue distribution must then be determined in reference to a multicompartment model. Despite the important information concerning the use of aminoglycosides in premature and full-term neonates provided by these investigations, they are – strictly speaking – so-called non-therapeutic studies and thus problematic from an ethical point of view. If ethical criteria had been strictly adhered to, these important data would never have been collected.

160

At this point, after the special aspects of pharmacokinetics, pharmacodynamics and toxicity in children had been presented and the necessity of incorporating special methods for determining drug effects and synthesizing drugs to meet specific paediatric requirements had been discussed, Reinhardt introduced the theme of ethical and legal problems of drug testing in children and asked Deutsch to give a short introductory speech.

Legal and Ethical Restraints

Deutsch first presented a brief historical synopsis of the development of the legal foundations of drug guidelines. He mentioned that in 1900 Prussian law referred to clinical studies in old and dying patients. It was the first time that so-called patient captive groups, which also included children, were taken into account. Deutsch then spoke about the 10 points of the Nuremberg Law, which expressly stated that in clinical drug testing the subject or patient must be capable of understanding the content of an experimental study, which automatically excluded children. He briefly dealt with the Declaration of Helsinki and the 2nd revised version drafted in 1975, which replaced the earlier declarations and the ruling of the Nuremberg military tribunal in the medical trials. It stated that studies in children – both for purely scientific as well as therapeutic purposes – are allowed when the legal guardian has given his or her "informed consent". In its most recent version this very general statement was expanded to the effect that the minor, when he or she is capable of understanding the content of the study, must be given a full explanation and must also provide his or her consent. This supports a general legislative trend whereby, under certain conditions, the child or young person must consent to the study. Deutsch then referred to article 40, par. 4, of the German Drug Act, which stipulates drug-testing guidelines. He pointed out that, in spite of the herein embodied intent to restrict studies in children, it is not clear whether these restrictions are meant to apply to both scientific and therapeutic studies. Legal precedents with respect to drug testing in children are extremely rare. Deutsch cited a 1975 California court decision involving studies in children under 2 years of age for which the parents of the children had received financial remuneration. In that court decision the judge referred only to a law concerning the prevention of crimes against children, but then clearly stated in his decision that, due to the existing loopholes in the law, investigations in children – including those which are not therapeutic – do not come under legal jurisdiction. Deutsch also called attention to a case which occurred several years ago in the Federal Republic of Germany, in which therapeutic drug monitoring had been carried out in children without the consent of their parents. At that time, a committee of experts from the German Research Association came to the decision that this study was necessary and not unethical. Despite the lack of legal grounds for evaluating drug testing in children, it is the general consensus that clinical trials in children must be kept to a minimum and the accompanying risk of side effects held as low as possible. At present, the general rule commonly adhered to is: therapeutic studies in children are only permitted when the risks are low, the parents have been informed and consent has been given. Whether this general definition applies only to therapeutic studies, or to non-therapeutic studies as well, has not, in Deutsch's opinion, been established.

Upon comparison of information from 13 European countries and 10 research centres in American Sereni pointed out the great variability in legal regulation and management of drug testing in children. While in the US the Federal Court is responsible for establishing guidelines for research in humans, this type of regulation is not in evidence everywhere in Europe, where only 9 of 13 countries have laws governing clinical research and only 4 countries have special laws concerning such research in children. He noted the large differences with respect to local commissions on ethics, which in terms of composition not only vary from country to country but also from hospital to hospital. In the United States, commission make-up is relatively uniform, with members of the medical profession in the minority. In contrast, in Europe physicians constitute a majority on such commissions. Both in the United States and Europe it is extremely rare that spokesmen for the parents of children in hospitals where studies are carried out are members of commissions on ethics. Sereni called attention to the fact that it is not possible for local commissions on ethics composed of physicians from these hospitals to make objective decisions regarding the research plans of their colleagues. He referred, however, to a statement made by Kennedy in Lancet in 1982: "The right of doctors to determine their own code of conduct has been generally accepted because they alone believe to have the technical knowledge to understand the issues". In addition to the issues of legal regulation in the various nations of the West and the variability in composition of local commissions on ethics, Sereni addressed the problem of "informed consent". It is generally agreed that for pharmacologic studies in children the informed consent of the parents must be obtained. But what presents a larger problem is defining when the informed consent of the child is necessary. In this context, differences exist between the United States and Europe: while in the US the consent of the child is generally called for, in Europe this is only true in part. However, a universal problem ist: when is a child old enough to provide informed consent. Inclusion of children in this information process creates difficulties because not only must the child be made to understand why, for example, a blood test is necessary but he or she must also understand the content of the study – particularly in the case of non-therapeutic studies. Sereni once again stressed the need for non-therapeutic studies as well and pointed out that all of the pharmacokinetic studies which have provided crucial information regarding age-related differences in the distribution and elimination of drugs were not directly related to improving the child's condition and thus actually come under the category of "non-therapeutic" studies.

The discussion then focussed on the issue of the clinico-pharmacologic relevance of experiments in animals, e.g., newborn rats and mice.

Boreus stated that animal models do not reflect the situation in humans and that experimental findings can scarcely be applied to clinical realities. Nevertheless, the process of development of a new drug must proceed from animal models. Boreus and Yaffe emphasized that the hitherto existing competition between experimental and clinical pharmacologic research for grants from research foundations must be done away with. Clinical drug research involves other methods and approaches and must, moreover, first and foremost, take the sick patient into account. Since no rivalry exists in terms of research content, there is no justification for it with regard to allocation of funds.

162

Hahn addressed the issue of investigations into the teratogenic effects of drugs and was of the opinion that here animal studies could prove valuable. Should such studies demonstrate teratogenicity for a substance, this would preclude its use in pregnant women. Yaffe replied that precisely teratogenic drug effects and studies designed to investigate these effects constitute a dilemma of sorts. Teratogenic effects in animals by no means signify that this is also the case in humans, and vice versa. One of the worst drug catastrophies, involving severe deformities in children born to mothers who had taken thalidomide during pregnancy, occurred because animal studies had failed.

Summary (Reinhardt)

Non-therapeutic, pharmacokinetic studies have provided great insight into the age-related criteria which determine the distribution and elimination of drugs. This has been significant in establishing dosage guidelines for different age groups. As yet, few studies have been done on pharmacodynamics, i.e., the interactions between drug and organism. It is therefore mandatory that future clinical drug testing include more pharmacodynamic studies than has hitherto been the case. It was pointed out that the developmental process in children involves a number of unique aspects, which necessitate the use of special methods for recording effects and monitoring treatment in pharmacodynamic investigations. A number of studies have shown that the response of the growing organism to drugs is, in part, quite different from that of the adult; this is also true with regard to the toxic effects of drugs. Thus the belief that in *every* case the younger organism, in particular the premature and full-term infant, is more sensitive, is not valid. In order to determine these unique patterns of interaction between drugs and the maturing organism, extensive, in part also costly, pharmacokinetic and pharmacodynamic drug studies – also those classified as non-therapeutic – must be carried out.

The competition between experimental and clinical pharmacologic research groups for research funds must be eliminated, since the questions asked in clinical pharmacology and the methods applied are quite different. Although the development of every new drug must begin with animal studies, these have very limited applicability in terms of clinically relevant issues in paediatric pharmacology. Clinicopharmacologic studies in children must therefore be more heavily supported than heretofore.

Despite data on age-related differences in pharmacokinetics and pharmacodynamics, the unique aspects of drug toxicity as well as specific paediatric disorders requiring specialized therapy, drug manufacturers have as yet shown little interest in paediatric concerns. Even for drugs already investigated in children only a few are available in presentations suitable for paediatric use.

Clinical drug trials in children are subject to certain legal and ethical restraints, which differ from country to country in the West. It must be required of every clinical study that it be scientifically sound, that the risk/benefit balance be acceptable and that the informed consent of the parents and also, in some cases, the young person be obtained. Furthermore, every study in children must be submitted to a local commission on ethics. The primary obstacle to carrying out clinical studies in children is, in most countries, the extreme vagueness of legal formulations regarding non-therapeutic studies and large differences in the make-up of local commissions on ethics and their interpretation of ethical guidelines.

All of the panel participants and members of the audience who took part in the closing discussion were in agreement that clinical studies in children are absolutely necessary. The fact that only a fraction of the drugs used in the different age groups has been investigated in clinical trials constitutes a dilemma for the physician involved in paediatric care. Organizations subsidizing research are strongly urged to support scientifically sound, clinically relevant research in the area of clinical pharmacology in paediatrics. Industry and pharmaceutical firms are called upon to take into account, independent of commercial interests, the unique aspects of drug therapy in childhood and to support both pharmacologic research and the development of suitable preparations for children.

The role of the EEC in the harmonisation of drug registration

C. A. Teijgeler

Introduction

The aim of the EEC is to obtain a free movement of goods and services within the Community. This aim also implies the free movement of medicines.
The EEC Treaty envisaged the free movement of medicines within the Community. This means that all barriers to the free movement of medicines should be removed. This aim has up to the present by no means been attained. In order to progress towards the free movement of proprietary medicinal products EEC directives have been drawn up to harmonize the legal provisions of individual member states, which have a direct bearing on the common market (article 100 of the EEC Treaty).

The directives

The first and most essential step was taken as early as 1965. The so-called *'First Directive'* defines in general terms the type of procedure which a member state has to follow when it considers applications for the marketing of new drugs, the standards which are applicable in respect to efficacy and safety and the periods of time alloted for the assessment of an application.
This directive has resulted in new national laws and in modifications of existing laws in the member states. The procedures currently in force for national drug registration are now the same in all member states. The criteria for the registration are standardized: "Authorization shall be refused if it proves that the proprietary medicinal product is harmful in the normal conditions of use, or that its therapeutic efficacy is lacking or is insufficiently substantiated by the applicant, or that its qualitative or quantitative composition is not as declared."
On the basis of these criteria it is in principle possible that in the member states the same new proprietary medicinal products are on the market, but on the contrary: there are differences! The interpretation of the criteria and the assessment of an application are different in the member states. The harmonization of national laws alone is insufficient to lead to a situation where all the regulatory agencies have the same attitude towards and the same results with drug regulatory practice. Moreover the historical background in the member states influences this practice by the authorities. After the First Directive which gives the basis for harmonization of the national laws, more steps are necessary. The EEC has taken a number of steps in order to reduce the disparities between the competent authorities of the member states. In 1975 two directives were introduced.
The *Third Directive,* 75/318/EEC, gives detailed specifications of the physico-chemical, biological and microbiological tests, toxicological and pharmacological tests and clini-

cal requirements to be met when a drug is licensed for marketing. This directive (the so-called Standards and Protocols) is a supplement to the First Directive, providing a clearer scientific basis for the contents of the application for a marketing authorization and for the competent authorities for their work on the assessment of an application.
More important is the *Second Directive* (75/319/EEC). This directive introduces the "Committee for Proprietary Medicinal Products", briefly known as CPMP.

The CPMP

In article 8 of this directive the purpose of setting up the CPMP is mentioned, namely: Facilitating the adoption of a common position by the member states with regard to decisions on the issuing of marketing authorizations and promoting thereby the free movement of proprietary medicinal products.

Three kinds of activities of the CPMP

1. An applicant has a marketing authorization (MA) in one member state and intends to place the product on the market in at least 5 (after November 1st, 1985, 2) other member states and one or more member states subject to MA.
2. Divergence of opinion of one or more member states (Commission) with regard to issuing, suspending or revoking a MA.
3. In specific cases where the interests of the Community are involved (for decision on a MA and so on).

In connection with these activities of the CPMP it is important to refer to the Council Directive of 26 October 1983, which amends the already mentioned directives.

Directive 83/570/EEC

This directive was based on the outcome of a series of discussions at Community level especially on "the mutual recognition of national licenses". This was proposed by the EEC Commission as the ultimate objective but the Council of Ministers was unable to reach agreement on this proposal. The aim of the Commission is mentioned in the Declaration of the Commission on the modification of article 15 of Directive 75/319/EEC (in 1983). This declaration runs as follows:
"The Commission considers the Directive 83/570/EEC as a step towards the objective of achieving the mutual recognition of marketing authorizations. The proposal which it will forward to the Council in application of article 15 will aim on the one hand at encouraging the adoption by the member states of a common position on applications for marketing authorizations and on the other hand at facilitating the recognition by the member states of authorizations already issued by a member state in accordance with Community directives."
This Council directive of 26 October 1983 amending the Directives 65/65/EEC, 75/318/EEC and 75/319/EEC on the aproximation of provisions is laid down by law; regulation or administrative action relating to proprietary medicinal products

(83/570/EEC) is very important. In the preamble is included that if in one member state a marketing authorization for a proprietary medicinal product is given on the basis of harmonized provision, this product will be allowed in another member state taking *into due consideration* the initial authorization.

The question can be put if in practice there is a difference between "mutual recognition" and "taking into due consideration". In general there are no big differences between the two terms if each competent authority has sufficient time to study the application and has its own responsibility to issue a marketing authorization and also the right to reject an application for a marketing authorization.

Having explained the aim of the free movement of medicaments attention will now be paid to the requirements of Directive 83/570/EEC.

Directive 83/570/EEC consists of the amendments and supplements to Directives 65/65/EEC, 75/318/EEC and 75/319/EEC relating to proprietary medicinal products.

Council Directive 83/570/EEC

Amendments and Supplements
65/65/EEC
75/318/EEC
75/319/EEC
The most important modifications of Directive 83/570/EEC relate to:
Directive 65/65/EEC
– summary of the product characteristics (data sheet)
  art. 4 b
  approved by the authorities
  art. 4 c
– adaption control methods after registration
  art. 9 a.
  accepted by the authorities
– expiry date in plain language
  art. 13.7
The new requirements in Directive 75/318/EEC (Standards and Protocols) are:

Council Directive 75/318/EEC

Standards and Protocols
– dissolution rate
– content active ingredient 95–105%
– mutagenicity studies obligatory for any new substance
– carcinogenicity studies' relation with mutagenicity
– bio-availability
In the Standards and Protocols Directive an attempt has been made to define the tests to be carried out and presented by the manufacturer. The *analytical* part of the Directive Standards and Protocols concerns the tests to be carried out on raw material, the production stage and the finished product. This analytical part of the directive is amplified with a paragraph on physico-chemical characteristics liable to affect bio-availability.

The *second* part of the Directive Standards and Protocols examines the different *pharmaco-toxicological* trials. A paragraph on mutagenesis has been amended. The study on mutagenicity is required for any new substance. The paragraph on "carcinogenic potential" is changed in relation to mutagenicity.

More important is the addition on bio-availability. In this part of the directive it is stated that for medicinal products which must be subjected to a bio-availability assessment, the data must include changes in the results as a function of time and, generally, indicate the bio-availability of the product or of its metabolites. The assessment of bio-availability must be undertaken in all cases where it is essential in the interest of patients, e.g. where the therapeutic safety index number is low or where the previous tests have revealed anomalies which may be related to variable absorption, or if this process is necessary for the proprietary medicinal products referred to in article 4 (8) of Directive 65/65/EEC.

This requirement is mentioned in the *third* part of the Directive 75/318/EEC. This part covers general indications for carrying out clinical trials and gives a basis for the investigations into applications for marketing authorizations for proprietary medicinal products on the requirements given in this part of the directive. The criteria to be used in evaluations are clearly described as follows.

"Evaluation of the application for marketing authorization shall be based on clinical pharmacological experiments designed to determine the therapeutic efficacy and safety of the product under normal conditions of use, having regard to the therapeutic indications for use in human beings. Therapeutic advantages must outweigh potential risks."

These provisions are of considerable importance in the EEC. On the one hand the applicant knows in general what data are required for registration and on the other hand the competent authorities in all countries receive the same data and can also reach the same assessment.

In connection with the requirements in the Directive Standards and Protocols there exist the *Notes for guidance* (Council Recommendation 83/571/EEC).

These notes for guidance have been drawn up by the Committee for Proprietary Medicinal Products (CPMP).

Their purpose is summarized in the preamble to the recommendation. The aim is that the Community Directives are used in the same way by investigators and by the competent authorities. Moreover there is a need for further information in order to avoid differences in assessment in the application of standards and protocols.

It should also be pointed out that the "Notes for guidance" signify progress in the field of harmonization, which is essential in the Community and which also assists in the recognition at international level of trials of drugs conducted in accordance with the notes, as well as helping to ensure that tests will not be duplicated when consideration is being given to export to third countries.

More details of the CPMP

In the second Council Directive (75/319/EEC), chapter III on the Committee for Proprietary Medicinal Products has been changed completely. The articles 8–15 have been replaced by new ones. In this chapter the procedure of the CPMP is described. The task of the CPMP is to facilitate the adoption of a common attitude by the member states with regard to decisions on the issuing of marketing authorizations and to promote thereby the free movement of proprietary medicinal products.

In order to realize a greater understanding between the authorities when files for marketing authorization are being examined and in order to assess in which direction to look for a solution to create a free circulation situation the CPMP had to express, in a limited number of cases, its opinion on the merits of drugs, i.e. their safety, their innocuity and their efficacy.

The Committee expresses its view in the following different kinds of cases.

– First of all on the request of a manufacturer wanting to export his product to at least five (after November 1st, 1985, two) other member states. If one or several of these five (in future two) other member states are not ready to grant the marketing authorization, the objections against granting must be examined and discussed by the CPMP which has to give its opinion within 60 days. The result of the discussion gives less objections than when all objections of the member states concerned are summarized. The opinion is not legally enforceable. An explanation of the new procedure is given (Fig. 1).

– The Committee can also express its opinion on a specific product on the initiative of a member state and without the intervention of a manufacturer. This is the case when there is a difference of opinion on whether a proprietary medicinal product is rightly

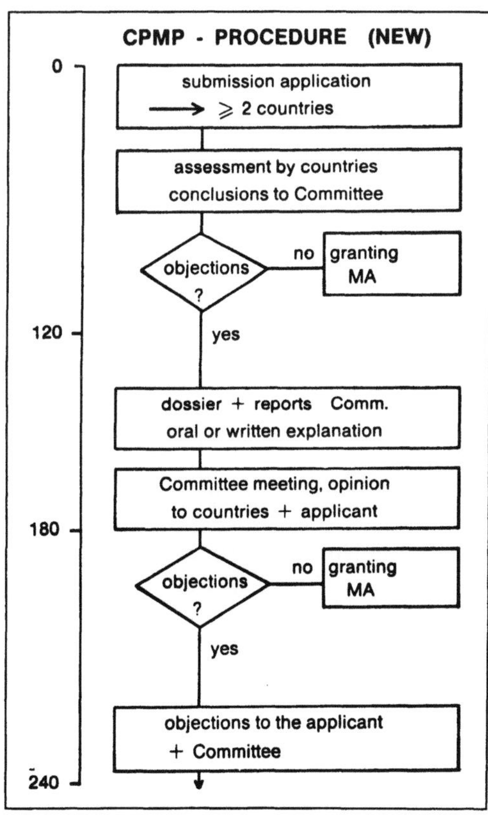

Fig. 1.

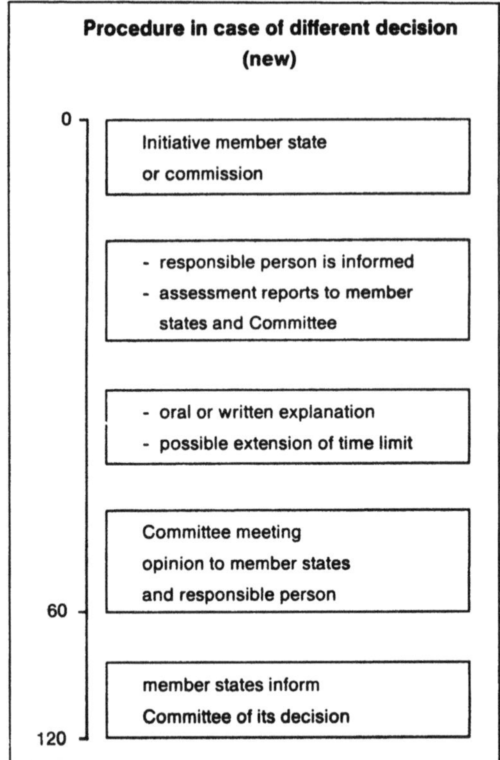

Fig. 2.

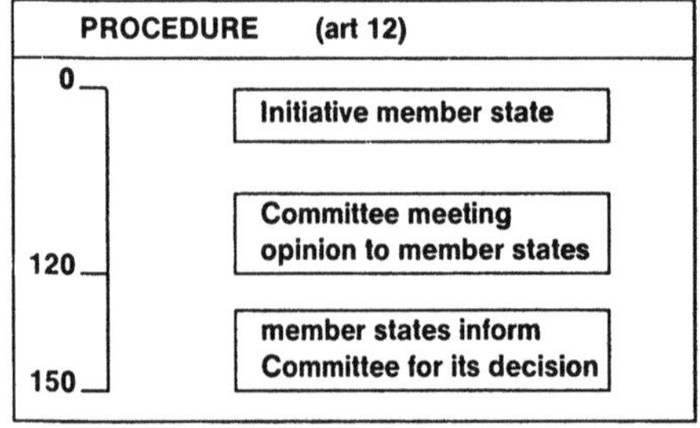

Fig. 3.

accepted or refused by another member state. From November 1st, 1985 the Commission of the EEC can take the same initiative. See Figure 2 for a scheme of the new procedure.

– If, for instance, a country perceives serious adverse reactions to a product marketed in that particular country, it can ask for the opinion of the members of the Committee and also for the opinion of the CPMP (Fig. 3).

The most important changes are:

– the competent authorities have to take an authorization issued in one member state in accordance with article 3 of Directive 65/65/EEC into due consideration.

170

- the person responsible for placing the product on the market has the possibility of requesting to explain himself orally or in writing before the Committee issues its opinion. In this situation the Committee has the possibility of extending the time limit.
- the Committee shall immediately inform the member state(s) concerned and the person responsible for placing the product on the market of its opinion or of the opinion of its members in case of divergent opinions.
- the Commission of the EEC has the right to refer questions to the Committee for application of the procedure referred to in article 14 of the directive. These questions are mentioned in the new article 11.
- the obligation to draw up an assessment report (article 13).

The assessment report must contain comments on the dossier as regards the results of the analytical and toxico-pharmacological tests on, and clinical trials of, any proprietary medicinal products containing a *new* active substance, which is the subject of a request for a first-time marketing authorization in the member states concerned. The assessment report should remain confidential and must be kept up to date (Fig. 4). The introduction of the assessment report in the CPMP procedure will be of great importance for reaching the same judgement on the same data. The assessment report plays an important role in the mutual recognition of the marketing authorizations in the member states.

The acceptance of Directive 83/570/EEC and Recommendation 83/571/EEC by the Council of Ministers is an important step forward in the direction of the free movement of proprietary medicinal products in Europe.

There is still a long way to go to achieve this aim, but if the competent authorities have the right attitude and goodwill, this aim will be reached in the future!

The role of the CPMP is also very important. The competent authorities of each member state should reach similar decisions based on the same criteria of quality, safety and efficacy. The CPMP aims at facilitating this and intends to take the following steps to reach this aim in the near future:

- the preparation of a guideline for drawing up assessment reports
- the assurance that no country authorizes a product without first obtaining an opinion from the CPMP. This is intended in particular to apply to medicaments developed using biotechnology
- the elimination of disparities in the assessment of individual medicines
- the anticipation of new developments
- assistance in re-evaluating old medicines

Assessment report

- report on the analytical, toxico-pharmacological and clinical data, submitted to obtain a MA
- includes comments and a critical judgement
- only for new substances
- shall remain confidential
- must be kept up to date

Fig. 4.

<table>
<tr><td>Proposal of the EEC Commission on "high-technology" medicinal products</td></tr>
<tr><td>

– In the case that the medicinal products are developed by means of new biotechnological processes each MS is *obliged* if it receives an application for a MA to ask an opinion of the CPMP

– In the case of other high-technology medical products the person responsible for placing the product on the market can *request* a MS to refer the matter to the CPMP for an opinion

</td></tr>
</table>

Fig. 5.

– the giving of opinions on the consequences of adverse reactions of medicines which are widely used in the Community.

New proposal of the Commission

In connection with these points the new proposal of the Commission is very important.
The Commission has made a proposal for a Council directive on medicinal products prepared by high-technology, particularly medicinal products derived from bio-technology.
The research of "high-technology" medicinal products requires a very long time and is very expensive. This research will continue in Europe only if identical conditions governing their placing throughout the Community are available in the near future.
The procedures in the present directives are not sufficient to open up to the high-technology medicinal products the large Community-wide single market which they require. Also the scientific expertise available to each of the national authorities is not always sufficient to solve the problems posed by high-technology medicinal products.
As a consequence of all elements the Commission has proposed a Community mechanism for concertation prior to any national decision relating to a high-technology medicinal product, with a view to arriving at uniform decisions throughout the Community.
As soon as the national authority receives an application for marketing authorization relating to a medicinal product developed by means of the new biotechnological processes which make use of genetic recombination hybridoma technology, e.g. aneuploid cell strains and enzyme bioreactors, the competent authorities shall be required to bring the matter before the CPMP for an opinion. This requirement shall also apply for other high technology medicinal products provided that the person responsible for placing the product on the market has expressly requested the competent authority concerned to refer the matter to the CPMP and has sent a copy of the request to the appropriate Committee. This procedure is optional (Fig. 5).
This important proposal of the Commission can be adopted following the advice of the European Parliament, the Economic and Social Committee and the Council of Ministers.
In the EEC there are more than 200 million people. The competent authorities of the member states, the EEC and the pharmaceutical industry have a great responsibility

for the health of the inhabitants of the Community. Close cooperation between registration authorities and the CPMP on one side and the pharmaceutical industry (EFPI) on the other is necessary.

Author's address:
Dr. pharm. C. A. Teijgeler
Chief Pharmaceutical Officer
Chairman of the
Committee for Proprietary Medicinal Products
Doktor Reijersstraat 10
NL-2260 AK Leidschendam
The Netherlands

Clinical trials – European recommendations

Jean-Michel Alexandre

Within the European Economic Community, the aim of the *Directives* is to bring nearer together the legal, regulatory and administrative requirements enforced in the member states. This harmonization is the first step necessary for the development of a registration procedure, either simplified within the Community (mutual recognition of marketing licences which at present is more of a myth than reality) or unified (community registration by a supranational authority).

To facilitate further this assimilation of the nationally enforced procedures and *technical* harmonization, started with the Directive 75/318 known as Norms and Protocols, the Committee of Pharmaceutical Specialities established two Working Groups to produce *Recommendations* (or *Explanatory Notes* or *Guidelines*):

– one, concerned with toxicological studies, known as the "Safety" Group and chaired until mid-1984 by Dr. Griffin (UK),
– the other, concerned with clinical trials, known as the "Therapeutic Efficacy" Group and which I have had the honour to chair in the last two years.

The subjects already dealt with and under discussion, the objectives of the Group, the procedures followed in production of its reports and documents, the status and the scope of the Notes are described below.

Subjects

The subjects dealt with by the Group and the points reached are presented in Table 1.

Objectives of the notes on clinical trials

The documents produced are the *Guidelines* for *Marketing Licence* applicants and their aim is to eliminate differences in interpretation while complying with the requirements of Directive 75/318 – hence the name *Explanatory Note* – in relation to relevant particulars of general nature (see notes 1, 6, 10, 11, 14, 15, 16, 17) or pertaining to individual therapeutic classes. For this purpose the Notes specify:

– *the essential grounds* which must be covered in the licence application dossiers; for instance in relation to drugs intended for oral administration the effect of food must be studied,
– *the minimal requirements;* for instance, safety assessment of drugs intended for long-term use necessitates presentation of high quality observations in at least 100 patients treated for 1 year,

Table 1. The various clinical recommendations and the levels reached.

No.	Title	Level reached
1	Specialized fixed associations	Text approved by the Council (recommendation CEE 83/571)
2	Cardiotonic glucosides	Documents approved by the Committee for Proprietary Medicinal Products (soon to be published as recommendations of the Council)
3	Oral contraceptives: clinical studies	
4	Oral contraceptives: notes for users	
5	Antimicrobial agents: notes for medical staffs	
6	Drugs for long-term use	
7	Non steroidal anti-inflammatory drugs	
8	Antiepileptic agents	
9	Drugs for chronic peripheral vascular diseases	
10	Bioavailability	
11	Pharmacokinetic studies in man	
12	Anti-angina drugs	Documents submitted for approval by the Committee for Proprietary Medicinal Products
13	Dermatological steroids	
14	General principles of clinical studies	In preparation
15	Trials in children	
16	Trials in the aged	
17	Sustained release preparations	
18	Antidepressants	
19	Anti-arrhythmic agents	
20	Drugs for cardiac insufficiency	
21	Drugs for cerebral insufficiency in the elderly	
22	Anticancerous agents	

— *the methodological approach* in general terms: the documents contain no technical details as they are not required by highly competent investigators and trial originators and would only be likely to interfere with their freedom of action and flexibility; for example, to provide objective evidence of anti-claudication activity it is advisable to recruit patients whose condition is stable, to verify its stability over a preliminary period of 4–6 weeks and then to evaluate the drug's efficacy not against haemodynamic criteria but on the basis of standardized effort tests.

Procedure for execution of recommendations

1. The subjects are selected on the basis of real *needs,* as perceived at the level of the Committee for Proprietary Medicinal Products and as presented by the Pharmaceutical Industry (represented by EFPIA).
2. Preliminary texts are prepared after *early consultation* with EFPIA, outlining the essential points (of the possible litigation) to be dealt with in the dossiers and seeking firm solutions to the arising problems.
3. Final drafts are then prepared by the Working Group assisted by experts.
4. These drafts are subsequently submitted for consideration by national agencies and industrial groups.

176

5. On the basis of the observations, comments and suggestions received the Working
   Group draws up the document proper.
6. The latter is submitted for approval by the Committee for Proprietary Medicinal
   Products.
7. The final documents must be approved by the Council before they are officially published as recommendations.

Status and scope of notes on clinical trials

On the conclusion of the process outlined above the Notes on clinical trials (as well as
those on toxicological studies) are published as recommendations of the Council.
The non-restrictive recommendations
– supplement the Directives (Directive 75/318 in particular)
– are intended for licence applicants in order to avoid litigation
– express the current scientific consensus
– are *unanimously* approved by the member states which undertake to enforce them
  and to follow them in the preparation of registration dossiers.
In practice, the recommendations
– should reflect the *needs,*
– should be *definite* and *brief,* limited to essentials, and must represent a genuine tool
  for the pharmaceutical industry and national agencies,
– should be published promptly for the information of interested parties (even at the
  project stage),
– should be periodically updated to reflect the progress of sicentific thought.

Conclusions

1. The recommendations which reflect the *Community position* on technical subjects are
   important, if not essential, as means to
– prevent errors and waste in the phases of clinical trials,
– draw closer together the scientific stance of member states and their representatives;
  the technical harmonization responding to Community needs facilitates the adoption
  of the increasingly desirable system of mutual recognition of licences and of the unified Community registration procedure.
2. Adoption of one or other of these systems of registration is one of the two essential
   preliminary steps on the way to free unrestricted circulation of drugs; the other being
   harmonization of the Community price and reimbursement systems.

Author's address:
Professor Jean-Michel Alexandre
Department of Pharmacology
Hôpital Broussais
96 rue Didot
75674 Paris Cedex 14 (France)

Discussion

The questions concerned the chances for realization of the EEC concept for simplification of the approval process:

1. Is it possible to use the same documentation for applications for approval in several member states?
This answered, "in principle, yes", since the EEC Directives have harmonized the contents and structure of the documentation to be submitted and the guidelines provide the basis for a commonly accepted interpretation. The necessity of updating when new information about the product has be gained through experience in the time between the first and later applications was stressed.

2. Are the guidelines for clinical testing of the EEC and WHO binding?
The member states of the EEC are obliged to follow the Directives of the EEC when they evaluate the documentation of applications for approval. The Guidelines are supplementary interpretations of the Directives for the various fields and are aimed primarily to be of help to the manufacturer in the testing of new drugs.
The Guidelines of the EEC were passed with the unanimous approval of their contents. Consensus was reached in three committees at three different levels; they can, therefore, be considered binding for all.
The WHO Guidelines, whose texts are scientific, are aimed to help physicians who want to study a medical problem in detail. Each is written by a small work group.

3. Can approvals in the other EEC states be expedited?
When a product has been approved in one member state according to the new laws, then an application for approval can be submitted
a) in another member state. The decision of this state must take due consideration of the decision of the first state or
b) in several other member states simultaneously through the community procedure of the EEC. The manufacturer's action is decisive since the effectiveness of the "new procedure" of the EEC in expediting the approval process is primarily dependent upon the manufacturer's use of this opportunity.

Panel discussion: international acceptance of data

Chairman: D. Poggiolini, Rome

Participants: J. M. Bilstad, Rockville
J. Drews, Basle
P. Fischer, Bern
R. Krebs, Wuppertal
G. Liebeswar, Vienna
H. Mandahl, Uppsala
A. Matsumura, Tokyo
B. Schnieders, Berlin
E. Snell, London

Introduction
D. Poggiolini, Rome

We can begin our panel on the international acceptance of data. You know that the problem of the acceptance of data, not only clinical, but all kinds of data, is of high interest around the world. In recent years most strict rules have been introduced in many countries for requirements for the proof of safety, the quality and efficacy of new drugs. The result of this request by regulatory agencies to the pharmaceutical manufacturers for more data for new drug applications is a progressive increase in the costs and time required for registration. We also have to consider that recently we have had a progressive reduction of new therapeutic innovations. On the other hand, we have also to consider that new chemical entities are so expensive that it is not possible for the pharmaceutical industry to introduce a new chemical for just one market.
A new chemical entity, today and in future years, must then result in a product for many markets. Thus the acceptance of data is a problem. But on the other hand we also have to consider the point of view of the regulatory authorities. We have to bear in mind that pharmaceutical regulatory procedures followed by various countries up to now have been generally based on autonomy in judgement and decision. This attitude was, in fact, based on the justified need to provide suitable safety for the respective population. In fact this resulted in a series of frequently repeated assessments on the same matter which were generally accompanied by requests for tests which had already been carried out elsewhere. It might be useful to consider whether these repetitions are really founded on scientific reason. This is the subject of our discussion.
I remember that the same problem has been treated in other meetings in other conferences, particulary in the Geneva conference in 1981 organized by the International Pharmaceutical Manufacturers Association. Now today we have a very good occasion to discuss the problem again because in this panel we have experts from different

areas: from the pharmaceutical industry and from the regulatory agencies. I think that each person should explain his point of view and in conclusion we can discuss the main topics deriving from the exposition of the problem.

Economical considerations
J. Drews, Basle

What I would like to do is to confront you with the economic impact of the heterogeneity of data and of the non-acceptance of data world-wide. I have taken the case of a multinationally operating company based in Switzerland. I could have taken one in Germany. The particular budget I am going to talk about is realistic; although the figures are not authorized they are authentic.

We will assume a research and development budget for all European cooperate operations for pharmaceuticals of 250 million Swiss Francs. Approximately half of that, 125 million, will be spent for clinical development, that is, not only clinical studies but all developmental work and all activities that have to do with the development of a compound from clinical phase I up to registration. Of these costs, 120 m Swiss Francs are divided between the three phases: 25 m are spent for twelve products which are in phase I; 50 m spent for approx. 4 products, in phase II; and 50 m are spent for only 1.5, on average, products in phase III (c.p.I). From this you can derive the annual cost of a c.p.I, c.p.II and c.p.III project, as I have done here. If you then multiply these various figures with the duration of each phase, then you arrive at the average actual cost for each successful compound: 102 m Sfrs. Now that will give you a registration dossier which will allow registration in Switzerland, Germany, Austria and perhaps in 15 other countries which do not have any strings attached, or claim not to have any attached, to their registration procedure with respect to the acceptance of foreign data. Now let us look at what you have to do in addition if you want to go into local national developments. There are two groups of member countries, of the IFPMA, one group has strings attached to the acceptance, but it claims to be able to work on foreign data alone. These countries usually require some clinical development. There are other countries where national studies are a must: one is the United States, one is Japan. There are some additional countries which play a minor role. I estimate the figure for an average development in phases II and III in the United States to be 25 m Sfrs, which is probably a modest figure; Japan with 12 m and five additional countries which insist on national studies and accept foreign data only as support material with 5 m. If you add that all up, you arrive at a total of 30 m Sfrs. If you then allow 2 m for each of the 15 countries with only very limited requirements for local studies, you have a total of about 72 m Sfrs. These figures are only estimated and could be plus or minus 10 or 20 per cent, but the additional expenses for the situation of the European-based companies, especially continentally European-based companies, is that an international development which allows marketing in about 15 other countries requires an additional cost of fifty to sometimes more than a hundred per cent. I think that when we talk about health expenses and the price for drug treatment, this is an order of magnitude which must certainly be considered and should play a role in our attempts to simplify matters.

Let me just give you a few very acceptable, from an industrial point of view, motivations for national studies. One is that there may be, and very often are, critical differences in patient populations, as has been mentioned a couple of times during this meeting. Secondly, there are differences in diagnostic categories, especially in areas like psychiatry which not only justify, but also warrant repetition of studies under somewhat different circumstances. There are also differences in therapeutical techniques and differences in therapy, for instance, the often cited example of peptic ulcer therapy in the United States and Europe. There are also cases where a confirmation of results through an identical protocol may be necessary. This may not be a complete list, but it gives you some idea of the motivations which would be acceptable to research-based pharmaceutical companies.

From the cost structure that I have presented to you and from the acceptable reasons for national developments, we have concluded that a very general umbrella that takes care of everything would not be a good solution. Rather, the solution should provide for the acceptance of a core document which can be supplemented by qualified specific studies in those countries where there is a specific problem.

Regulations and Reality
R. Krebs, Wuppertal

To continue the line of Professor Drews, I would like to add that if you divide the total R & D budget into research and development, then you will certainly see that there is a shift away from basic research toward development. This is in spite of the fact that we always officially talk about and agree upon some "common procedures", some acceptance of data. There is no doubt a trend towards acceptance, but on the other hand, the development costs are increasing. We now have only 30 per cent for research in our company. If we extrapolate that to the year 2001, we will no longer have any research; all the money would be needed for development.

Why is this all happening? I think opinion is divided on this. Usually we talk about the ideal situation. Everybody officially agrees upon that. The problem is that there is an unofficial procedure. If, for example, you go to a registration authority which has an agreement with other countries, you certainly will find that the medical review officers who have to deal with the practical questions do not know the general agreement or do not follow it.

In France, for example, it is not officially necessary to repeat analytical work. But in practice? You have an expert agrée who has to write a report for the authorities. But when you show him the data he will certainly repeat some of your work because he says – sometimes rightly – "I have to convince myself in my lab.". So he repeats the work in spite of the fact that it is officially not necessary. This is the kind of thing we have to watch, because it increases costs in spite of our general policy of acceptance of data.

This also occurs when a pharmaceutical company applies for clinical trial permission or for an approval. Some countries then send written statements of what you should do additionally. In some of the countries it is possible to arrange meetings to discuss those critical issues and if you have a meeting usually you come to an agreement on the work still to be done, which is less than when the issues are not discussed since misunderstandings can be cleared up. I would very much favor the introduction of a hearing like that proposed in the last session of this conference, so that we can discuss whether results are really lacking or whether there is a misunderstanding.

The differences we have in Europe also reflect national differences which are not yet covered by any agreement between the E.C. countries or the E.F.T.A countries. For example, if you apply for clinical trial permission in Italy, you have to submit five mutagenicity tests instead of three in the other E.C. countries, and you have to use two species in six months, which is more or less unique in Europe. This is just for clinical trial permission, not for the application.

If safety is really improved from such tests, it would be alright. We all agree on that. But then the question is: why do other countries not need these tests for clinical trial permission?

I have not included Japan in this discussion because the difficult procedure in Japan will be presented later on and should be discussed then.

Appraisal of directives
E. Snell, London

In addition to the important question of cost and delay caused by duplication of effort – animals and patients are of course limited and precious resources – there are also very important ethical considerations. Although with respect to patients this has been discussed quite a bit during this conference, especially with regard to children, we have not yet touched on the question of the ethics with the use of animals. As you all know the animal welfare movement is strong and gaining attention around the world in varying degrees. The Council of Europe will soon be adopting a new convention on this that will probably accelerate legislation around the world. It has certainly already provoked legislation in the U.K. where we shall soon have a new bill for the use of animal experimentation. This we cannot ignore. Let us now turn from that to the needs for the reciprocal acceptance of data required to avoid that unethical, unnecessary and costly waste. The data, of course, must be of assured quality. We need some means of verifying this.

The amount of data required must be agreed upon by mutual agreement on its content. We must get the most we can out of all of this work with these precious resources.

Now let me just deal with the preclinical and the clinical aspects of this work, firstly pointing out some important differences between the animal work and the human work. The animal work is indirect, the really interesting thing is the toxicity in humans and it is hoped that the animals will predict that. This is fairly standardised type of work, basically the same whatever the type of compound or drug and largely empirical. In contrast, clinical work is direct, it gives you the answer you want: what happens to patients. The way this work is conducted is tremendously varied in nature. Furthermore, a third party does this work: the clinician, who takes responsibility, and has his own views and his own independence to consider. In new fields of therapy where the industry is engaged in pioneering activity, there is no precedence to go by.

Now let us look at these two aspects, the preclinical work first. Good laboratory practice is now generally used for the assurance of the quality of the data for this preclinical work. In the U.K. manufacturers have also accepted the F.D.A. rules and the F.D.A. inspectors when they want their data to be accepted in the States. But we have got a problem ahead: if we want reciprocal acceptance of good laboratory practice standards we need to avoid multiple inspections and multiple different systems. The O.E.C.D. guidelines on this seem to be close to those of the F.D.A. and industry fields are adequate to form a common pattern for general acceptance. In the U.K. the government has worked out a national scheme for verifying data that is being used for Japan.

Guidelines for preclinical work are necessary but they do have dangers. They can, if made too rigid and too much of a check-list, obstruct the progress of toxicology. In the first part of this conference, it was made quite clear that toxicologists are developing some intelligent techniques which will allow experimentation to find its own way rather than just follow a check-list. The preparation of guidelines requires full consultation with toxicological experts in the industry. Great flexibility must be provided in their construction, in their implementation, and their assessment. The O.E.C.D. guidelines are not appropriate for this purpose; these were drawn up for chemicals such as pesticides and agricultural chemicals and are not, we feel, suitable for pharmaceuticals. There are plenty of other GMP guidelines for pharmaceuticals. The C.P.M.P. guideline is fully accepted by the industry, but if the companies try to get their products marketed internationally, then they may have to consider other guidelines. The sooner we can get some reciprocity of acceptance of the same standards of work throughout the world, the sooner companies can really limit their work. Otherwise the companies always have to do the most that anybody wants anywhere in the world.

The assurance of the quality of clinical data has not been discussed very much. We heard a bit about Good Clinical Practice in the States, where they seem to need such guidelines, and in Japan, but I do not think there is any great interest in the U.K. or in the E.E.C. The clinical guidelines, as presented in Professor Alexandre's very nice contribution, can be fully agreed with and accepted by industry as long as the whole situation works out as quickly and neatly as Professor Alexandre has suggested. Past history with such guidelines, I am afraid, has not been so happy. We have had them in extraordinarily different lengths, without consultation.

Industry feels that there is a need for one general clinical trials guideline, and that the others can be very short, almost as short as Professor Alexandre's slide, which seemed to be a prototype of what a guideline should be. They should not be like the WHO documents. You do not need, once you set down general principles in a guideline, to keep repeating things about ethics and numbers and statistics as is done in the WHO guidelines. Number 14 on Professor Alexandre's list of guidelines seems to be the kind of general guideline which we have proposed to the E.E.C. for some time.

Industry favors the acceptance of common guidelines and common submissions in the European Community. It is willing to accept the efficacy guidelines as long as these directives promote agreement, which they seem to do. It was very interesting to hear Dr. Teijgeler's account of the proposed new directives, which seem very laudable. But we have to consider one danger: we in industry fear that an F.D.A.-like authority could arise over Europe and put industry into the sort of situation they have in the States. We hope that the national authorities will hold on to their national responsibility, and that mutual acceptance will never – or at least for not for a long time – become automatic and mandatory, but always remain subject to review by a competent national authority. The proposed new system for high technology products makes reference to the C.P.M.P. mandatory for the first time. Our industry has accepted this so far in order to support agreement among national agencies, but there is a danger here that mandatory reference to the C.P.M.P. could very easily be extended. The list of products could be lengthened and so we would end up referring everything to a supernational C.P.M.P. I am sure this will not happen, but I would like to draw attention to this possibility.

Evaluation reports – experience by E.F.T.A.
P. Fischer, Bern

After the signing of the first Pharmaceutical Agreement in the E.F.T.A. – the Pharmaceutical Inspection Convention – and agreement for mutual recognition of inspections among countries, a Work Group in the E.F.T.A. was created in order to initiate harmonization in another area. We have observed that among the agencies in the E.F.T.A. countries, there is a strongly felt desire that each agency know about the decisions of the others and the reasons for the decisions, for example, why an approval was not granted but also why it was granted. The goal was actually – I guess you can say it this way – a double one: that the agencies come not only to a harmonization in the area of Good Manufacturing Practice, but also in the area of "Good Registration Practice" and especially "Good Evaluation Practice".

The instrument envisioned was a simple exchange of Evaluation Reports (on the documentation submitted by the manufacturer among the agencies) according to the well-known E.F.T.A. principle: internationally – pragmatic – the harmonization of the national evaluations.

A second point: the agreement should be open. The official exchange is not limited to E.F.T.A. states. A basis prerequisite should be achieved, if possible: the manufacturer's documentation which is submitted to the various agencies involved should be identical. The longer our experience with this, the more this requirement seems necessary.

Furthermore, summaries should be included which contain self-evaluations for the clinical part, the pre-clinical part, etc. with references to the original documentation. The reports on the results of pharmaceutical, pharmacological/toxicological or clinical investigations should be written by experts and contain evaluative conclusions on the assessment of quality, efficacy, and safety of the product.

These were, more or less, the goals. Let me say that we were aware that the path would be rocky because of the large burdens which would fall to the agencies. Our first evaluatcpn report included no less that 60 pages; it was, for the receiver, a useless instrument. The second consisted of 30 pages – still far too many. We then decided that the goal should be no more than 15 pages. We are now working in various work groups on attaining this goal.

Difficulties are created not only by the extent of the material, in the necessity of receiving the identical documentation from the manufacturer so that the other agencies can judge on the basis of the same information, but also in providing for the appropriate consideration of the positive elements of the national evaluation. This is because – and we in Switzerland are not alone in this – the reports of the evaluations tend to consider only the negative consideration and say nothing about the positive elements since this is simply not considered necessary. In an Evaluation Report, however, the consideration of the relative benefits and risks is absolutely necessary.

The Evaluation Report serves another purpose, and that is to avoid repetitions as far as possible. The information submitted forms the basis for the evaluation.

Two things have already been achieved: one is that the idea that an evaluation report should be written and then exchanged has somehow attracted attention, it has somehow worked as a motor – a promoter. We observe this with great satisfaction, even though the realization of the idea still lags a bit behind expections. And then, the second: we hope, and are convinced that the E.F.T.A. system can becpme effective in many states through multilateral agreements. In the pharmaceutical field, only agreements which are bilaterally executed are usually considered practicable. A classical example of a multilateral system which was proven effective on a large scale is the Pharmaceutical Inspections Convention. What we have done until now with the exchange of Evaluation Reports goes beyond the bilateral level and has proven effective as a system. We hope that we can depend upon the cooperation of the manufacturers since the system certainly makes cooperation between the agency and the manufacturer as well as among the agencies easier.

Common guidelines – Scandinavian proposals
H. Mandahl, Uppsala

We are really discussing two different things here first, the acceptance of international data as a part of a new drug application and, second, exchange of information between registration authorities. I would like to comment a little on both. First, as far as Sweden is concerned, the question of the acceptance of foreign data in the new drug application is very simple. We accept all data, regardless of the origin of the data; the only thing that matters is the quality of data. This is, of course, a very simple way of expressing things. In practice we have rather hard requirements on the quality. Things that are regarded to be of good quality in some parts of Europe or some parts of the world are not necessarily regarded as being of good quality in Sweden. We do not, in principle, ask for any duplication of work or investigations. We have had situations when we have been convinced or have suspected that the data given to us did not really give us a full picture of the drug or the group of drugs. In those cases we have asked for additional data performed in Sweden. This was the case a number of years ago with MAO inhibitors, and I would say that the situation today with fixed combinations of beta blockers and diuretics is about the same. We still ought to have some typical Swedish information about the usefulness of these drugs.

Also, in cases where ethnic differences might occur, we are interested to find out whether the drug is specially suited for the Swedish market. In general, we accept all data provided that the quality is acceptable to us.

The second item is the exchange of data between authorities. I would like to present some of the work the Nordic countries have done in this field in the hope that this will provide useful ideas for the E.F.T.A. and E.C.

Our idea and the idea brought up by Professor Drews is that there should be some sort of common guideline or common base for work which, later on, will end up in some kind of exchange. In the Nordic countries we have worked out common Nordic guidelines in a number of areas.

The first guideline covered allergen preparations. This was a rather easy area, because none of the countries had any guidelines. We had no traditions and we had no prestige in this field.

The second one was somewhat more a matter of dispute, but it has been accepted by all the Nordic countries. The last one, which will come into force in the Nordic countries at the latest on the 1st of January next year, took us a lot of time to write. Industry was involved and their views were taken into consideration in this work. This guideline is compatible with, and arranged in the order of the E.E.C. directive. This is an attempt to create a bridge to the E.E.C.

The second step in this future system is that the new drug applications be arranged and the information required by the common guidelines be organized in the order we want it, so that we know that we have the same documentation. We have seen from studies that industry is not sending the same documentation to all countries. Also the documentations are not sent at the same time.

The next step after evaluation is to prepare an evaluation report or assessment report, as Dr. Teijgeler named it. Work on this is now going on in all three communities: we have heard about the assessment report in the European Community and we know from Dr. Fischer that the E.F.T.A. is preparing one. The Nordic countries are also in the process of establishing the outline of an evaluation report. I have the same hope that Dr. Schnieders has that we will have one common, exchangeable evaluation report outline for all European countries. Work on this will take 6 months, 10 months or more. It is very important for the three groups, the Nordic, the E.F.T.A., the E.E.C., to come close together in this field.

Finally, I would say that as we know from the Nordic experience, when we have something to exchange among the Drug Regulatory Authorities and it can be put to use, that is when the real problem starts. Because we then have a system, we will be accused of not using it effectively enough. There are a lot of obstacles in the evaluation procedure: attitudes, administrative procedures, different ways of communicating with the manufacturer, confidentiality – all these obstacles must be identified and removed.

Evaluation reports – the Austrian View
G. Liebeswar, Vienna

As the third member of the E.F.T.A. family I would like to continue with the question: what role do Evaluation Reports, which can be requested, play in the approval process? I think that when we have answered this question, we will come to the conclusion that the PER Scheme, which Austria welcomes, will be a transition phase.

In Austria, and certainly also in many other nations, we follow the principle of "free proof" for regulatory processes. This means that for the approval process these reports must be considered as evidence just as all other data and evaluation reports available to the agency. The staff member confronted with all this material must primarily ask the question, the very simple but therefore very difficult question, what is the real situation. This means that he must consider the principle of material truth: that is, he must study the documents with the same absence of bias that we expect of a scientist.

A pharmacologist, for example, does not agree with an opinion just because it is expressed in the textbook edited by Goodman and Gilman. If, for example, another pharmacologist can show that he has obtained results different from those in this text book, and if this colleague works carefully, and if he can even show why he got results different from those considered to be correct, then the evaluator will more readily accept the results of this investigator than those in the textbook. The staff member must work in a similar manner: he must orient himself on the quality of the data and the evaluation reports received by the agency.

One additional consideration seems to be of great importance in the Austrian administrational process. We recognize the principle of thrift: the principle that the process must be carried out as simply and quickly as possible. This principle requires us to take the considerations that Professor Drews presented at the beginning of our discussion especially seriously. In other words, in the future, the health agency will have to consider the cost-effectiveness of its measures for drug safety more carefully. I think that therefore, this transitionary measure, which is certainly not now fully satisfactory, can lead to considerable progress.

Evaluation report: structure and contents
B. Schnieders, Berlin

In all cooperation systems the Evaluation Report plays an important role: the Nordic Council, the E.F.T.A., (the P.E.R. Scheme) and the E.C. What is the real purpose of these Reports?
The first purpose is certainly to make optimal use of the documentation submitted by the manufacturer for approval of a new drug. This is certainly an advantage for the manufacturers.
The second purpose is to make optimal use of the evaluation reached after the assessment of the documentation as well as the judgement on the documentation as proof of efficacy, safety, and quality. This is certainly an advantage for the agencies.
An Evaluation Report must be written in the future for all new substances the first time they are subject to an application for approval.
We have already said much about the advantages of the Evaluation Report. What are its contents, how is it organized, what is the present status of the discussion on it? The scientific basis for the report is the documentation submitted by the manufacturer: the dossier. The summary evaluations (Expert reports prepared by the applicant) required for the documentation are very important. These summary evaluations and the conclusions on the pharmaceutical, pharmacological and clinical properties of the product as well as the general evaluation of the benefits and risks of the product form the basis for the Evaluation Report. These summaries are not then re-written by the agency as was the original practice but are used directly as first part of the report. The quality of these summaries is decisive for the Evaluation Reports, since the second part of the report contains the agency's critical opinion of the summary. These critical opinions comment on all parts of the documentation submitted, including the results and conclusions. The same or different conclusions can be drawn from the data, and the lack of important data is noted.
In the third part, the official decision of the agency is explained. The reasons for the decision are stated. Why was the decision made the way it was – not only positively, but also negatively. Furthermore, a complete description is given of the decision itself – what does the licence say, what is in the product description, and under which conditions can the product be placed on the market.
Finally, a bibliography must be attached which lists the documents on which the evaluation was based. Also, when much time has elapsed between the first evaluation and the application under consideration, we must consider updating the report with a follow-up report which contains the experience with the product in practice, both positive and negative.
At present, we are trying to gain agreement among the organizations mentioned on the structure and contents of evaluation reports so that they will be compatible and the same reports can be used in all the member states of all the organizations involved.
Let me just add the following: when we speak about acceptance of clinical documen-

tation and acceptance of foreign data, we are referring not only to positive data, but also to negative data, not only information on successful therapies, but also on unwanted effects.

One important aspect of this was already hinted at: the completeness of the documentation submitted. Documentation has not always been as complete as required and necessary for the agency's evaluation. When, for example, after examining the cases of side effects reported in an application, one reads in a Lancet article published the year before about many cases which were not reported in the application, one must consider whether paragraph 96.6 of the Drug Law has been disregarded. This paragraph requires the manufacturer to submit complete documentation and provides for legal punishment for non-compliance.

In summary we must then ask the manufacturers for their help – in their own interests – with

1. the summary evaluation in the documentation for the application for approval and
2. the completeness of the information in the documentation.

so that we can work optimally and efficiently.

Acceptability of foreign clinical studies by the F.D.A.
J. M. Bilstad, Rockville

My comments will cover only the acceptance of foreign clinical studies. Certainly the F.D.A.'s position has evolved over the years to one of greater acceptance and reliance in foreign studies. In part, this probably reflects some evolution in design and conduct of clinical studies throughout the world and the submission of higher quality clinical data. As scientific standards for the clinical study of drugs gain wider acceptance throughout the world, unnecessary duplication of clinical studies becomes more clearly unjustifiable. The F.D.A. advised the pharmaceutical industry in the 1960s that foreign clinical data meeting the standards of adequate and well-controlled studies would be acceptable, but it was not until 1975 that a formal policy on foreign clinical studies was incorporated into the investigative new drug regulations. These regulations remain in effect today. The conditions outlined must be met if foreign studies are to be used in support of a new drug application. Basically they cover four areas: sponsors are to verify that the investigators are well qualified by training and experience, that the investigators have adequate facilities, that the investigators maintain detailed records and that these are available to the sponsor upon the F.D.A.'s request, and fourth that the studies are conducted under acceptable ethical standards for protection of human subjects. I mentioned previously that the F.D.A.'s position has evolved over the years to one of greater acceptance. The 1975 regulations stated that foreign studies could be used to support approval of a drug for marketing, but that the agency has generally also required that some clinical studies be performed by an investigator within the United States. Such a statement is included in the New Drug Application Form and the only exception noted is the situation in which the disease for which the drug is being used is so rare in the United States that testing is impractical. In 1982 the F.D.A. proposed major changes in the N.D.A. regulations. Even though these regulations have not been accepted in final form, it is worth noting that they signal a further evolution in policy toward data derived from foreign clinical trials. The introductory section clearly

188

expresses the policy that all clinical studies are to be considered under merits, regardless of the country of origin.

The proposed changes greatly expand the circumstances in which a new drug application can be based solely on foreign studies. All such applications are to be considered on a case by case basis.

There are three general conditions that were spelt out in these proposed regulations.

The first relates to the applicability of the foreign data to the U.S. population in medical practice. As has been mentioned previously, there may be medical, genetic and cultural differences among countries which dictate whether or not the findings from one country can be extrapolated to another. Some drugs are metabolized at different rates by different populations.

In addition, cultural differences may affect certain diagnoses, particularly in the psychiatric area, and frequently concomitant medications given during clinical trials vary considerably.

The second condition for approval of an application based solely on foreign data is that the studies be performed by clinical investigators of recognized competence. The F.D.A. can verify the qualifications of a clinical investigator in the United States, but it cannot verify the qualifications of many foreign investigators.

Factors that might be considered in judging the competence of a foreign investigator include, for example, an international reputation, experience in evaluation of drugs, and publications in well- known scientific journals.

The third condition for approval of an application based only on foreign data is the judgment that the data can be considered valid without the need for on-site inspection by the F.D.A. or, if the F.D.A. considers such an inspection to be necessary, that the agency is able to validate the data through an on-site inspection or another appropriate means.

The F.D.A. can obviously conduct only a small number of on-site inspections of investigations of foreign clinical studies, in part because our resources are limited, and in some cases because such inspections are nor permitted. To date the agency has attempted to conduct on-site inspections in only a few countries. Given the limitations in the number of inspections that can be conducted by the F.D.A., drug sponsors are strongly encouraged, where possible, to verify the validity of information submitted to the agency through their own on-site audits of medical records.

If a sponsor is considering submitting an application based only on foreign clinical studies to the F.D.A., we urge early consultation between the sponsor and the agency before the application is submitted. There are some situations in which the F.D.A. would consider foreign studies more likely to provide the sole basis for approval. Examples include a drug that results in a major health gain or a drug for a disease that is uncommon in the United States. A drug that has a very favorable benefit to risk analysis would also be considered a likely candidate.

While the F.D.A. expresses the policy that new drug applications can be based solely on foreign clinical data, the agency also believes that such applications will be relatively uncommon. In fact, the agency very strongly encourages drug sponsors to conduct at least some studies in the United States. Sometimes these studies may help to settle more specific issues of labeling; sometimes they may determine whether a lower dosage can be used; sometimes they may make a better outline of pediatric indications in recommendations for dosages.

How would I evaluate clinical studies that have been submitted to support new drug applications recently? It is my impression, and that of most of the F.D.A. reviewers to whom I have posed that question, that the overall quality of foreign studies has been improving in recent years. This impression applies primarily to studies in which the drug sponsors have participated directly in the design of the protocols and have monitored the studies. On the other hand, studies in which the drug sponsors have not been directly involved frequently contain flaws in design and possibly also in conductor reporting results. This severely limits the weight that the F.D.A. gives to such studies.

These limitations apply particularly to foreign clinical data that a U.S. sponsor has purchased under a licencing agreement. The studies are not only more frequently of lower quality, but also in this situation, the foreign manufacturer has no obligation under U.S. law to supply complete or accurate information to the licencee. The licencee also usually has had no direct contact with the clinical investigators.

The reliability of adverse drug reaction reporting in foreign clinical trials is obviously highly dependent on the care with which the clinical investigator monitors the patients during the course of the study. When the monitoring procedure is adequate and the details are clearly spelt out in the study report, the F.D.A. reviewers feel assured about the validity of the adverse reaction reporting. But when such details are lacking, little weight can usually be given to the safety findings, particularly when few adverse reactions are reported.

In conclusion I would like to emphasize the following points: first – all clinical studies will be considered by the FDA on their merits regardless of the country of origin; and second – there are certain situations in which the F.D.A. will consider accepting only foreign data in support of an N.D.A., although we believe such applications will be uncommon, and we encourage drug sponsors to conduct at least some studies in the U.S.

Acceptability of foreign data – the Japanese position
A. Matsumura, Tokyo

I would like to explain the position of the Japanese government concerning the acceptability of foreign data in the field of drug licencing.

Recently there has been increasing demand for the rationalisation and simplification of the drug approval system as a means of opening up the Japanese market. In view of such circumstances, and in an effort to eliminate unnecessary duplication of studies, the Minister of Health and Welfare has endeavored to expand the scope of the foreign data which can be accepted.

At present, policy on the acceptance of foreign data in Japan is, in general, as follows:
First of all, all foreign data concerning physiochemical properties, standards and test methods of imported drugs shall be accepted.
Stability data is required for

- long-term stability
- stability under severe conditions
- acceleration tests.

Foreign stability data can be now accepted. The standards for stability data were amended extensively last June to allow pharmaceutical companies to submit the final long-term stability data at the time of approval rather than in the initial New Drug Ap-

190

plication submission, if long-term stability of the drug is expected. The new drug application can be accepted provided that:

- the data of the severe test and the accelerated test suggest relatively long-term stability;
- long-term stability data for more than one year are already available.

Secondly, toxicity data are most important for the evaluation of drug safety. The Minister of Health and Welfare decided in March 1982 to accept foreign toxicity test data provided that:

- the studies have been conducted in conformity with good laboratory practice;
- the studies meet the toxicity test guidelines of Japan.

Before this change was made, animal test data used by foreign governments for evaluation could be submitted if accompanied by a certificate given by the authorities of the country stating that these data had been used for evaluation of the drug.
One important matter in regard to toxicity studies is the evaluation of test methods. The Minister of Health and Welfare promulgated the notification on "Guidelines for Toxicity Study Methods" in February 1984, in response to a request form the E.C.
These guidelines include the methods for general toxicity studies and methods for special studies such as those for carcinogenicity, reproduction, mutagenicity, etc.
Thirdly, data from studies on pharmacology and on absorption, distribution, metabolism and excretion conducted in foreign countries are accepted.
All preclinical data are now acceptable. We are still discussing acceptability of clinical data with people in Japan and with people in other countries.
In the case of preclinical studies, the evaluation of study methods and reliability of data are important for the acceptance of foreign data. For clinical data, genetic differences and differences in medical care and nutrition and diagnostic standards between Japan and foreign countries must also be considered. Therefore at present foreign clinical data are handled as follows.
Data from phase I trials conducted in foreign countries in Japanese nationals will be accepted as data for new drug applications. Of course, these studies should be carried out with appropriate procedures and methods (for instance they must be conducted in accordance with the regulations for clinical trials in the country of origin and conducted in accordance with the standards for clinical trials in Japan).
When the plan for the phase II clinical trials is submitted in accordance with the provisions of the Pharmaceutical Affairs Law, the results of the phase I trial must also be submitted, noting that the phase I clinical trial was conducted using appropriate procedures and methods. Foreign phase II and phase III trial data can be accepted as supplementary data in Japan, but the core data must come from clinical trials conducted in Japan.
In the submission of foreign preclinical and clinical data the following points must be considered:

- the data must be scientifically sufficient to allow evaluation of the quality, efficacy and safety of the drug;
- the data must be prepared by reliable personnel at reliable institutions.

In order to make these requirements clear, the Minister of Health and Welfare has prepared guidelines for study methods, especially study methods to ensure the safety of drugs, and established G.L.P.'s for tests. These have made the acceptance of foreign data possible for almost all preclinical tests.

However, two problems still remain, the first being the acceptance of foreign clinical test data in Japan, and the second the harmonization of guidelines for test methods among countries.

As mentioned previously, foreign data from phase II and phase III clinical trials can be used as reference data. We do pay attention to them, but clinical data from tests performed in Japan are required as core data.

Foreign data may be accepted for phase I, if the tests are performed in Japanese nationals. The Minister of Health and Welfare (MHW) is now being requested to accept clinical data from studies in foreigners.

Summary
D. Poggiolini, Rome

In summary, we can say that progress has been made in Europe in the following areas:

1. The mutual recognition of documentation, based on the guidelines of the Nordic Council and the E.C.
2. The development of the community procedure. The same elements, for example, the evaluation reports, are a part of the P.E.R. Scheme and the E.C. community procedure.
3. The harmonization of the evaluation report. The aims are to produce common requirements for the official evaluation report and to make its contents and structure the same for both the P.E.R. and E.C. systems.

The new information from the USA on the acceptance of foreign clinical data and from Japan on the acceptance of pre-clinical data sound very good.

It is clear that the requirement for supplementary studies in France mentioned by Professor Krebs in his talk belong to an out-dated administrative measure. Such a general requirement would not concur with the European Directives.

A question about the quality of clinical studies done in Latin America, Portugal and Spain and their information value could not be answered because of the lack of experience. In the USA a few studies have been submitted, some were considered good, some were considered not so good, especially in their design.

The necessity of the harmonization of requirements and for cooperation – especially among the E.F.T.A. and E.C. states – in the field of drug safety is unquestioned. The question about an eventual supranational agency was answered, in summary, as follows: the efforts to create similar requirements for the scientific documentation for applications and to create the same form for the Evaluation Reports which have to be written for new substances in the E.C. and P.E.R. systems as well as to use these reports for each specific decision are seen as cooperative measures and not as supranational measures. Only the national agency can be responsible for the final decision on the approval or rejection of an application since this agency bears the responsibility for the health of the people it serves.

In spite of this, savings of time and money can result from the common efforts of the P.E.R. and E.C. for both the manufacturer and the agency

– through avoidance of repeated studies and evaluations,
– through the common recognition of documentations,
– through the general consideration of the benefit-risk assessment in the Evaluation Reports.

The legal situation allows a reduction of waste through cooperation and the national agencies realize the necessity of taking advantage of the opportunity to reduce waste. Sceptics are reminded of the example of the European Pharmacopoeia which is now a reality.

The Japanese authorities accept phase I studies carried out in a foreign country when these are properly carried out with Japanese subjects. Another question about a further acceptance of foreign studies – for example of phase II studies – was answered negatively. Japan does not presently see any possibility of accepting other clinical data. It is, however, in a phase of scientific discussion whose end has not yet been reached.

Let us close the discussion with the wish that in future international congresses of physicians in the pharmaceutical industry, a detailed and critical report on international developments in the acceptance of foreign data be included as a special topic on the agenda.

The Pharmaceutical Industry –
research and responsibility

Hansgeorg Gareis

K. Oppenheimer said that physics lost its innocence with the explosion of the atom bomb.

When the splitting of the atom was successfully achieved in Göttingen, the way to the bomb but also to the greatest source of energy ever was opened up. The application of the results of experimental research had changed the world.

This is of course an extreme situation. But extreme situations are often useful for posing a basic question: namely the question of the responsibility of research.

What is the responsibility of research? We must consider this question afresh every day because it has become a matter of life and death.

I should therefore like to define the field of research in very broad terms: from clinical research to scientific research in the laboratory, and further to research into the Arts. Anyone who is engaged in any form of research today will be confronted with these questions at some time. And he will have to give an answer if he wants to take his place among thinking people.

It is certainly right to establish first of all what research actually is so that we can proceed from a common point.

What does research do? It looks for the new, the hitherto unknown. In doing so it follows a basic human instinct: curiosity. The eros of research is the attempt to satisfy this curiosity.

Man has always used all the resources available to him to satisfy this urge. Even the myths of classical antiquity were obsessed with the dream to fly. The Tower of Babel was to be high enough to reach the sky. Columbus risked life and limb to reach the unknown land of spices and to prove at the same time that the earth is round; the force of fire was used to conquer distances more rapidly with a machine, the train. But also Immanuel Kant, Martin Luther, Karl Marx, Karl Jaspers and Martin Heidegger searched for the new and posed the question about truth.

So is research, the search for the new, really only a means of satisfying the curiosity instinct?

What does research do?

Research looks for new experiences, for more knowledge. It tries to improve and optimize that which already exists. It tries to achieve what we call progress. Research seeks to advance. No progress is possible without research.

Deputy member of the Board of Management of Hoechst Aktiengesellschaft, Frankfurt/Main

The work of the research scientist is summed up by Bert Brecht's Galileo as follows:
'Indeed, we shall question everything, everything living again. And we shall not advance in seven-league boots but at a snail's pace. And the discoveries we make today we shall dismiss tomorrow and shall not reinstate them until we have rediscovered them. And once we have found what we are looking for, we shall regard it with particular mistrust. Our observation of the sun will therefore go hand in hand with the unwavering resolution to prove that the Earth stands still. And only when we have failed, are completely and utterly beaten and are licking our wounds, shall we begin to ask in the depths of despair whether we were not right after all and the Earth does rotate. But should every theory except this one prove to be false, there will be no mercy for those who have not done their research and yet hold forth.'

When we regard research in such terms, it is something quite basic; something that can change the conditions under which we live. People who are involved in research have a responsibility. They cannot merely follow the urge to satisfy their curiosity.

The major responsibility of those who are engaged in science, the scientist or the researcher, is for the knowledge they have acquired to be reliable. The society of researchers and society as a whole expect what the scientist finds and then say to be true to withstand examination. And even if there is only a slight suspicion that results have been claimed which will not stand up to investigation by others, the author may be excluded from scientific circles.

To find the truth and only the truth is the first responsibility of the scientist, today as it was a thousand years ago.

The researcher is part of society

Despite this extraordinary demand made on his activities the researcher, as part of society, cannot claim to be something special, an outsider. In the community at large the researcher is also a part of the whole.

In the communities in mediaeval towns every citizen was responsible for the general welfare. He had to place himself and his activities at the service of the community. Only then would the community look after him in return and protect him from enemies and other trouble. Without this protection he would have been at the mercy of thieves; without this protection his house would have burnt down because he was not in a position to put out the fire himself.

Today's pluralistic society is divided up to a far greater extent than was society in the mediaeval town. Craftsmen have developed into highly technological and highly specialized professions. Only by such professional differentiation is it possible to manufacture and develop products which meet our stringent requirements. Once a standard of living has been attained, constant development, continual improvement of the goods is required if it is to be maintained.

In this pluralistic society the researcher takes on the responsibility of further development, innovation. Without him the goods produced would soon become uninteresting, and town and state would eventually sink into insignificance. Because others would have taken on the task of innovation and would make better, more interesting products available.

But on the other hand with the high degree of specialization of our sciences the individual researcher is no longer able to earn his living as well as pursuing his own lines of

196

investigation, searching for the new. Research has become a means of living, a profession. The researcher is dependent on the fact that society provides him with a living.
The researcher is therefore part of the whole because society enables him to devote himself entirely to the search for the new. Of course it demands a quid pro quo. It expects this return service in the form of excellent research achievements and results.
The responsibility increases. Not only do scientific circles expect genuine results that withstand examination; society as such expects results which are beneficial to everyone. The urge to satisfy the curiosity or to satisfy personal ambition is by no means enough for an understanding of science itself.

The benefits of research

But who can be great enough, you could almost say omniscient enough to be able to distinguish between that which is beneficial to society and that which is not.
Was the discovery that the nucleus of the uranium atom can be split beneficial, was the development of a machine for the artificial resuscitation of humans beneficial, or wasn't it? Was the development of highly effective antibiotics a good thing or has it largely contributed to the overpopulation of the earth?
We all know that in the case of Galileo the Rome authorities, in those days the all-powerful church authorities, assumed full responsibility. They forced the scientist to recant two of his important statements. They compelled him to confess that what he had found did not correspond to the facts and was therefore not true.
The Catholic church had decided in 1633 that it was more beneficial for society to regard not the Copernican conception of the world as the truth but that the stars revolve round the Earth. The Earth stands still; it is the centre of the universe.
It was not the Earth's rotation as such that disturbed the church. It was the fact that an important religious dogma had been questioned. The dogma stated: the Earth is the centre of the universe and man, God's image, stands on it. Everything moves round the stationary Earth. Anyone who doubted this dogma was shaking one of the major pillars of the faith and therefore questioning the credibility of the church itself. Every past belief would totter.
In retrospect we can see how wise and foreseeing it was. The danger was not the recognition of the solar system as such but the consequences this discovery would have.
Of course the silence that was imposed on Galileo was only beneficial for a few years. Galileo's scientific experiments and observations established facts and after only a relatively few years these results were made known despite the ecclesiastical decree banning the Copernican theory. Consideration of these facts called a conception of the world into question. By questioning the dogma that the world is the centre of the universe, systems of thought and philosophies were changed. Brecht's Galileo said: 'That which has been believed for 1000 years is now the subject of doubt.'
However, in my view, we must also realize that not only scientific or medical experiments can have extraordinary consequences. Ideas and philosophies can have just as far-reaching results. Jesus Christ and Buddha changed the world but Immanual Kant and Karl Marx changed thought processes and the way of life with their new systems of thought. Science and research cannot only be regarded in scientific terms, but must be considered on a broader basis – the humanities must be included.

The question of who should assume the responsibility for new discoveries is more urgent and more far-reaching due to the broad basis on which we have now seen and defined research.

Belief in and fear of progress

Our forbears would have never or only rarely posed such questions. At the end of the 19th century in the preindustrial age and certainly up to 6 August 1945, the date of the first atomic explosion over Hiroshima, questions of sense and non-sense, of responsibility for new knowledge were largely unknown. New machines had relieved some of the drudgery of work; new methods had provided food for an increasing population; new drugs had eradicated the epidemics that had for centuries been the scourge of mankind. A material standard of living, which would have been inconceivable a few generations before, had been attained. New systems of thought had been established which gave large sections of the population a mental and physical freedom which had hitherto never been known in the history of mankind. The new, that which had come from science and research, progress, had become beneficial to all mankind.
Nevertheless, today, at the end of the 20th century, the concept of progress still carries a ring of doubt; indeed the question must be answered: is or can progress be dangerous, perhaps even undesirable?

How could there be such a radical change in the attitude to progress?

Until August 1945 all that could be achieved by research was immediately apparent, changed very little. That which science could change, changed nothing fundamental. Galileo's experiments and these explained natural phenomena, but did not change them. Of course they changed man's conception of the world; but they did not change the processes in the natural world.
It can now be said that the change in man's conception of the world altered human thinking fundamentally and there is no more radical change than this. But hasn't the thinking of a Martin Luther or a Karl Marx effected a tremendous change? Haven't these two men changed entire epochs for instance and ushered in new ones?
In theory, however, it would be quite possible to think that anyone more powerful would have revised Luther's and Marx's ideas and therefore the consequences would have been different, or even that these ideas would have remained without consequence.
But an atom bomb explosion is irreversible and can never be undone. Nuclear fission is an irreversible fact. The fact that man has created living conditions under which the human race is increasing in leaps and bounds cannot be undone – it is an inescapable fact.
Everything that man was capable of doing in the past could be reversed by nature. His buildings could fall down; wounds inflicted by wars could heal again and everything artificial that had been made by human hand could be absorbed into nature again.
Man has now complied with the text from the Bible: he has made nature his subordinate.

This is the new situation: man has acquired a power which he has never before had in his history. His power seems to have extended beyond the point where he can control it himself. Even he finds it almost inconceivable. In this new situation, which has never existed before, man is beginning to fear himself. For this power can never be taken from him again, by anyone, except himself. He himself will have to change to remain master of the authority he enjoys.

Research as an activity in the creation of the new

Progress, to all intents and purposes, has some if not the major share in this new dimension.
In addition to the authority, which already existed, recent years have brought the possibility of intervening in hereditary information. Genetic engineering came into being.
In 1956 Watson and Cricks postulated that genetic information consists of nucleotide sequences and is arranged in the chromosome in the form of a double helix. Later it was found that the information can be transmitted from one organism to another and that this transmitted information is recognized and read off by the recipient organism. It had become possible to make a genetic change and therefore intervene in evolution. We are learning to recognize the limits which have perhaps been imposed on man by nature itself in this field.

Is it therefore surprising that there are doubts as to whether much of what man can do today is beneficial and right?

In addition there is the fact that our scientific structure has now become so differentiated that even experts often have trouble understanding the finer points of an allied field. How much more difficult it is to make factual knowledge in a specialized field comprehensible to the layman, even the willing layman. And it is particularly the incomprehensible, the mysterious that causes concern, causes anxiety.
Our concept of responsibility has therefore become wider. In addition to finding the truth itself it is a responsibility to society to ensure that the possible application of what has been discovered is beneficial. Such a responsibility can only be met however by discussion. And a discussion, a conversation, in which two sides take part, is only possible if the participants understand each other or are willing to learn to understand each other. Research has therefore been driven out of its ivory tower because it has to seek contact, approval from the outside world.

Can research be stopped?

It should of course be said that anyone who becomes nervous in a strange house should best find the quickest way to get out of this house, to leave it as soon as possible. We could therefore say we shall call a halt to, even forbid, research, because then no damage can be done. It would be the easiest way; but is it feasible?
I should like to answer this question, even in the light of what has been said so far, with a categoric 'no'.

We know that in 15 or 20 years' time at least 5 or 6 thousand million people will be living on this earth. In cities such as Calcutta, Mexico and São Paulo 30 million people will be living in one place: the mothers who will bear these people have already been born and nothing, apart from perhaps an atomic disaster on a worldwide scale, can prevent the birth of these thousands of millions. Who could maintain in all seriousness that these people will be able to live in woods and green fields? There have never been, and there never will be, that many woods and fields on this earth. In view of this population problem alone, i.e. without any other forces which may also exist, it is not possible to call a halt. On the contrary there is an urgent need for changes and innovation in order at least to attempt to find a solution to this tremendous problem.

We have therefore got ourselves into a predicament from which there is no way out other than forward. It is no longer possible to go back: we passed the point of no return long ago. We do not even know where it was: It is as in a difficult mountain climb, where the way back has become so dangerous that the only option is to go on with great care because this is the only way of reaching the refuge.

But it is necessary for us to be aware of our predicament and not delude ourselves that we have an alternative to pressing on, which would enable us to reach our refuge more safely or even turn back.

So does this mean: continuing as before and merely trying to put the danger behind us as soon as possible?

I am afraid we shall not be able to live without the danger any longer: it will constantly accompany us, like the chorus in Classical Greek drama. As in Classical Greek drama the chorus, in its role as commentator and admonisher, was the constant companion. And perhaps that is a good thing. A constant reminder that the way is fraught with danger can be helpful.

We must now widen the circle still further: Research bears the responsibility, as we said before, but in the knowledge that survival is only possible if we go on and the way ahead is fraught with danger.

There is nothing new in the fact that going ahead, making progress, is hazardous. Every time we take a new path we encounter the unknown: otherwise the path would not be new. And the unknown can always mean either: good or evil. We should know in good time from our experience whether on the new path a crevasse is going to open up or an unclimbable precipice or perhaps a by-way which will finally take us to the top.

Responsibility towards whom?

The great responsibility of research, ultimately, for the possible survival of society is more complicated.

It affects people in an age in which many of them have cast almost everything overboard: the existence of God is in question; the concept of morality has at best given way to a set of morals which an individual recognizes for himself; coexistence can only be controlled by national laws because other restrictions no longer apply. The almost boundless freedom into which man was cast after the Age of Enlightenment and the technical development in this century has deprived him of supports for which he has found no substitute.

In this situation the question of responsibility to whom is much more difficult to answer than we may have thought at the outset.

There are cases where our question is easier to answer because it is much more obvious: An airline pilot in his cockpit is responsible for his passengers. They sit behind him and he can see them when he leaves his cockpit and walks through the cabin. They rely completely on him and are entirely dependent on him. It is his responsibility to deliver them safely to their planned destination.

In most situations it is also easy for the doctor to define his responsibility: he should restore the health of his patient or at least try to reduce suffering. He committed himself to this when he took the Hippocratic oath.

It is more difficult to define the responsibility of the researcher. Should he answer to society of which he is a part, should he answer within the framework of his own ethics which should determine his actions or should he be answerable to God?

The Christian researcher must obey the Commandments: he must be aware of the consequences of his actions, what is permitted in his faith and what is not.

For the researcher who is not a believer it is very much more difficult to define the area of responsibility. 'Après moi le déluge' and 'I shan't be around to see it' are sayings which are heard from time to time. But this word 'flood' carries more weight now than ever before. Because it has become reality. As we shall very soon know, we can create a flood with all our bombs. And the final account, when everything has been destroyed, is of no interest because the last great judgment seems to be no longer possible.

However when the researcher feels that he is part of the whole, his responsibility can only be to the whole, and that is society. He cannot say, like Brecht's Galileo 'As scientists, it is not up to us to ask where the truth will lead us.' He cannot climb the difficult mountain on his own. His rope party can also be not only scientific society because this, like he himself, is only a part of the whole. His area of responsibility can only be society as a whole. It enables him to make the climb and expects from him, and that is the great responsibility, a climb that will lead as safely as possible to the difficult goal. Anyone who has ever been in a rope party will know that a slip or carelessness on the part of one person puts the whole group at risk. The responsibility of the individual is linked firmly with the group and therefore with the whole. One cannot live without the other.

The question which we posed above, namely that of the great man who should know what leads to good or evil can, at the end of the 20th century, probably only be answered as follows; 'In a fair discussion in which each partner recognizes the constraints but also the knowledge of the other, the way must be found between research and society which will finally lead to the goal.'

An answer therefore which will certainly not satisfy all of us but which I can only express in this way. However, such an answer, when it is given by both partners with conviction and in the same terms requires the same degree of commitment and the same responsibility from both partners. Not only the scientist can feel responsible: society must feel equally committed. But at the same time this means that society must inform itself, or be kept informed, of the facts.

When a hearing in the Bundestag, the Lower House of the West German Parliament, on genetic engineering reveals complete ignorance on the part of the questioner (and members of the Bundestag are after all representatives of society, of the people), one is of course doubtful about the sense and outcome of a discussion. When fellow citizens, and Greens are fellow citizens, are not prepared to find out enough about the constraints that are placed on our society, a discussion is not possible.

If industry and government eventually reach a consensus on a way ahead, we cannot address ourselves to the problems involved unless a discussion is possible. There is a great risk that we shall not reach the top. The extent and consequences of this risk are immense.

Can responsibility inhibit creativity?

For the purpose of our reflections here, however, let us assume that the discussion is possible and proceed on the assumption that research, the individual researcher and society as such are prepared to take on the responsibility. Can the impact of the extent of the responsibility inhibit the researcher; can it add to the difficulty of the research activities?

I think that that may be the case but I would hesitate to say that it is bound to be. Not only for the researcher is it necessary constantly to monitor his position. Even a conscientious airline pilot continually checks his position despite all the instruments that are at his disposal.

But I will not deny that many people approach an experiment more hesitantly, but maybe also more deliberately, than they would if they were not aware of this responsibility.

It is however an old and strict rule that no experiment should be carried out unless the result can, with great probability, provide the answers to a clear-cut question. This in no way rules out the possibility that a planned experiment may produce an answer different from that expected. But the question must be clear-cut and the experiment must be such that an answer can at least be expected.

If this prerequisite was observed, many of the premonitions of science critics would be unfounded: because only those experiments would be carried out which were planned in such a way that a clear-cut answer could be expected. But it would also mean that experiments which are irresponsible would not be performed.

But there is of course also the question whether the constraints that are imposed by such a responsibility can impair creativity. Creativity is the result of imaginative thinking, the search for new paths. The researcher who, on realizing that he is on the wrong track, has to look for new, different possibilities, can be regarded as creative.

I think that discussion, as we understand it here, would not be a barrier, but on the contrary an incentive, even a compulsion to creativity. In discussion it was decided early on that when the path becomes uneven, maybe dangerous, when the compulsion becomes recognizable, new and different paths must be found.

Freedom in responsibility

The sheer extent of the responsibility is bound to lead us to the question of the freedom that still remains in research after all that has been said. It was Johann Gottlieb Fichte who demanded it most urgently. In a scientific memoir which he delivered to the public in 1793, he said 'Free investigation of every possible object of consideration, in every possible direction and into the unlimited, is without doubt a human right.' And our German constitution states: 'Art and science, research and teaching, are free.' But at the same time it states: 'The freedom of teaching does not absolve one from loyalty to the constitution.'

Above we discussed the question whether, at the end of the 20th century, man can or should do everything for which he has the facilities at his disposal.

Just as Fichte demanded in 1793 we know today that research requires freedom. Without a large measure of freedom, without the possibility of taking a gamble, effective decisions cannot be made and creativity cannot thrive. It would be absurd to want to dictate to the laboratory researcher which experiments he must carry out. Interesting pieces of news often come from the unforeseen result of an experiment. Chance, the unconventional idea, is essential for successful research work.

And yet: Monitoring of the researcher, restriction of the freedom of research work by any authority at all?

Expressed in these concrete terms it is a contradiction to the dogma that no good research findings can be obtained without freedom.

With a few exceptions a researcher is constantly being monitored. He has to write reports which are monitored as an assessment of his work. In many cases the resources at his disposal depend on this assessment and on the objectives of his work. This applies both to research at the universities and Max-Planck societies, as well as in industry.

Freedom is already restricted in research activities as it is everywhere else. Our interdependence compels us to recognize limits and controls. If I expect the State to protect me, I must also be prepared to show the guardian of public order my credentials if he wants to see them.

Planning research objectives?

The researcher is part of the whole, one of the players in the game. His freedom, like that of others, is restricted by the fact that the results of his work are investigated.

But is he free to choose how to approach his work, free to decide which field he will work in when he has to justify his results?

Shouldn't there instead be a scientific plan to prevent, right from the outset, undesirable results from being obtained?

Research in a free society must be free also in the choice of its goals. The free play of forces ensures of its own accord and very efficiently that the forces of research are concentrated in areas where results which are important and useful for future work are to be expected. Central planning in research is as futile as it is in the economy. There are several large-scale projects which a state or even an association of states should and must finance. There are projects of this type in nuclear physics: there are also some when particular lines of research are activated, for instance in genetic engineering. A state should promote projects and stimulate lines of work, but it must not restrict or limit the freedom of research.

Only discussion can apportion responsibility

So where is the way out of the dilemma? Research requires freedom and creativity. But at the same time it has become such a powerful instrument that its results can cause anxiety, even fear. However, the constraints which are imposed on us make research and its results the prerequisite of our survival. But a 'world research control' is impossible.

There is no solution other than discussion between research and society. A discussion of course, which must be held honestly and openly by both sides. Both partners must realize that they are dependent on each other. It is not that only one can bear the responsibility and give the other the change of saying 'It was your fault'. Galileo's results could be recanted for a while. But of course only for a very short time. That is where the Roman Klerus went wrong: occasional recantation does not solve the problem.

Then as now it must be realized that once something has been learnt it cannot be unlearnt. If Galileo had not looked through the telescope, somebody else would have done, if Otto Hahn had not carried out his experiments somebody else would have discovered the splitting of the atom and if Luther had not ushered in a new era, somebody else would have done. When the time is ripe for a discovery, it will be made.

Prohibition is not the answer; instead the knowledge gained should be examined in a responsible manner.

The problems facing us can only be solved by discussion and therefore with joint responsibility. And the problems of present and coming generations are extraordinary.

Let us try honest and open discussion. There is no other way.

Commemorative paper given at the award ceremony for the Paul-Martini-Prize 1984, in Munich on October 17, 1984.

Author's address:
Hansgeorg Gareis
c/o Hoechst Aktiengesellschaft,
Postfach 80 03 20,
6230 Frankfurt/Main 80
F.R.G.

Subject Index